The Overweight Child

Promoting Fitness and Self-Esteem

The Overweight Child

Promoting Fitness and Self-Esteem

Teresa Pitman and Miriam Kaufman, M.D.

FIREFLY BOOKS

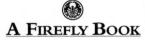

A FIREFLY BOOK

Published by Firefly Books Ltd. 2000

First Printing 2000

Cataloging-in-Publication Data
Pitman, Teresa
      The overweight child: promoting fitness and self-esteem /
Teresa Pitman and Miriam Kaufman. –2nd ed.
[   ] p. : cm.

Originally published under title: All Shapes and Sizes : Toronto :
HarperCollins, 1994.
Includes bibliographic references and index.
ISBN 1-55209-474-X

1. Obesity in children – Nutritional aspects. 2. Obesity in Children –
Psychological aspects.
3. Child rearing 4. Body image in adolescence. I. Kaufman, Miriam. II. Title.
613-7042   -dc21   2000   CIP

Published in the United States in 2000 by
Firefly Books (U.S.) Inc.
P.O. Box 1338, Ellicott Station
Buffalo, New York, USA
14205

Design by Interrobang Graphic Design Inc.
Printed and bound in Canada by Friesens, Altona, Manitoba

Canadä

The Publisher acknowledges the financial support of the Government of Canada through the Book Publishing Industry Development Program for its publishing activities.

For Reg.
And
for Roberta, who loved me
even when I was having an
affair with my laptop computer.

Contents

Acknowledgments

Many people provided help, support and encouragement in the writing of this book. We'd like to thank, in particular, The Hospital for Sick Children for giving us access to its research library and computer; Sharon McKay for putting us together in the first place; Anne Day; Sandy Pearson; Joanne Tee for her help with the sections on teasing and self-esteem; Riziero, Andrea and Alyssa Vertolli who took care of the children while Teresa went on a research binge; Lenore Kilmartin; Lesley Hennin for her patience during the last week before the manuscript was due; the entire Cherrywood community for their support at a time when there was little energy to spare; our editors, Susan Broadhurst, Fran Fearnley and Dan Liebman; and, of course, our families who helped to test out the recipes and offered their own special kind of encouragement.

Introduction

Come and sit with us on a bench outside an elementary school and watch the kids arriving on this spring morning. It's warm enough today that some of them are wearing shorts instead of track pants; some are walking, some are riding bikes, some are dropped off by their parents. We have a mixture of ethnic backgrounds here, and you can hear parents saying good-bye in several different languages.

I can guarantee you that you'll also notice, if you watch for a little while, that children come in different shapes and sizes. See that group of seventh and eighth grade kids hanging around the baseball diamond? Some of the girls have been through puberty and are almost at their adult height; a few of the boys are tall, too, but most of them haven't yet had that growth spurt and they look surprisingly short beside the girls in their class.

And now watch this group of girls walking into the schoolyard. Three of them are wearing shorts and T-shirts; the fourth is dressed in sweatpants and a loose sweater. It's obvious why, too: she's fatter than her friends, and even though she probably feels the heat more than they do, her desire to cover her body is stronger than her need to feel comfortable.

She isn't the only child her size at this school. If you keep watching, you'll see many more – and you'll notice some larger-than-average parents, too. Just as any group of ten-year-olds will include some short ones, some tall ones and many in between, so children will range from thin to fat.

The difference is that because of societal prejudices, being a fat child is a much more negative and painful experience than being a tall or short one. And it can be almost as painful for the parent who watches his or her child struggle against teasing from others, with the resulting damage to self-esteem. Parents worry, too, that the child will suffer serious health problems as a result of his or her weight.

If you are the parent of one of those children, we hope in this book to offer you reassurance, solid information and practical suggestions.

One of the things that has made this book difficult to write is the lack of neutral terms to describe the larger-than-average child. A smaller-than-average child can be slim, slender, slight, petite – even thin or waif-like has positive connotations in today's society. But how do you write about the heavier child when every word that might be used has such strong negative connotations? Just listen to them – fat, overweight, obese, heavy, chubby, husky.… Would you like to be described with any of those words? We remember hearing one child say that she was "fat-and-ugly" as though it were all one word. In addition, character traits are often linked to weight – lazy, lacking willpower, slovenly, stupid. The words that refer to overweight are all ugly words.

So how can we discuss this problem without a more neutral word to use? We've chosen, for the most part, to use "overweight" even though we don't like the connotations behind it – that there is some perfect, ideal weight that every person of a certain height should achieve. We have plenty of research to share with you to show how wrong that concept is. But "overweight" seems to us to carry less of the intense negative baggage than other words like "fat" and "heavy."

Our society is obsessed with weight and body size. This pre-occupation is a serious problem. In a *Chatelaine* article on women's obsessions with thinness, the author, Suanne Kelman, interviews Jackqueline Hope, who is 5′7″ and weighs 190 pounds. Hope feels comfortable and healthy at that weight and says, "I knew I was over-weight but I really liked my body, and I couldn't understand why other people didn't. It was a pretty, Rubenesque body and it was mine, and I couldn't understand the hatred I would feel for it once I started to diet."

Then Kelman comments: "No matter how hard I try, I can't understand Hope's celebration of her 190 pounds of flesh. The thought of anyone parading nude in front of a mirror at 190 pounds literally makes me gag."

We find those comments terrifying. How can a larger-than-average child develop self-esteem and a feeling of being uncon-ditionally loved when the society around her – and probably even her parents – finds her size so repulsive and disgusting?

People justify their bias against heavier children and adults by saying that weighing more than average is unhealthy. But the link between weight and health continues to be tenuous. Some researchers have suggested that it is repeated dieting that causes health problems for overweight people, and that those risks are much lower for those who maintain a consistent weight even if it is higher than average. Certainly, if your child is extremely over-weight and you feel that there are health problems because of this (such as difficulty breathing or skin infections) you should speak to your doctor.

But there are many other unhealthy aspects of our lives that don't cause such strong emotional reactions. Would the author of the *Chatelaine* article write, "The thought of someone getting a sun-tan literally makes me gag?" In fact, tanning – clearly demonstrated to be unhealthy – is generally accepted and tolerated. Friends may encourage heavy sunbathers to modify their behavior, or express concern, but they don't feel disgusted or repulsed. Fat phobia is clearly based on something less rational than health issues.

If you walk through any art gallery and look at art through the ages, you can see that the idea of what constitutes an attractive body shape changes from era to era. Even fifty years ago, the ideal body shape was more rounded than it is today. And different cultures have different preferences regarding body shape and size.

All of us are susceptible to anti-fat biases. It can be difficult to find a physician who will make a realistic overall evaluation of an overweight child's health and not focus solely on his or her weight. In research studies, teachers have been shown to have more negative feelings about heavier students and to perceive them as "lazy."

It's also difficult for parents. If your child is larger than average and you are also struggling with your own weight, you may feel both guilt and anger. Did your child learn bad eating habits from you? Is his weight your fault – just like yours is? And thin parents may find it impossible to understand why the child doesn't just lose weight. It seems like such an easy task for them. One divorced father told his daughter, who had begun to "fill out" as puberty approached, "You're going to end up fat just like your mother." Yes, he intended that comment to hurt his ex-wife, but it was also very painful for his daughter.

People often excuse these hurtful comments by saying they make them for the child's own good. They hope to shame or embarrass the child into losing weight. In fact, they tend to have exactly the opposite effect. Only by demonstrating genuine love for your child – whatever her size – will you be able to help her work towards increased fitness. Overweight children can be just as attractive, loving, kind, intelligent and lovable as any other child, and they need to have that confirmed on a regular basis. Living with a constant assumption that there is something wrong with who you are (such as your body size) leads to low self-esteem. This, in turn, can lead to lowered self-expectations and therefore lower levels of performance, in school, sports and socially.

If you, the adult reader, are also overweight, you may be surprised by some of the new research presented in this book. The problems of low self-esteem, feeling disgusted with yourself and enduring teasing or criticism from others may be all too familiar.

However, if you have been through many cycles of dieting and weight loss, you might be expecting a recommended low-calorie diet for your child. You won't find that here because dieting doesn't work, not for adults and not for children. What you will find are ideas for changes that can help your entire family become fitter.

Weight and body size are far more than a health issue. In our society today, they are very emotional topics. We hope this book will help you get past any negative feelings and raise your child to be happy, confident and fit, no matter what his or her body size may be.

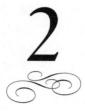

The Truth about Being Overweight

Are you concerned about your child's weight? Have others commented that he or she is getting chubby? How can you know if there is a problem – if this is really something to worry about?

The Dangers of Being Overweight

Is being overweight a major health problem? We've been convinced by our society that it is. But let's look at some of the research.

In his book *Lifespan*, Thomas J. Moore looks at the life insurance tables that have become popular standards for weight. He notes that the "ideal" weight is that at which people have the longest life expectancy, and that at weights below and above that ideal, people will die earlier. The more overweight (or, of course, the more underweight) the person is, the greater the risk of premature death.

However, on closer examination, the risks are actually quite modest. A man who weighs 20 percent over his ideal weight at age 45 has a loss in life expectancy of 3.6 months. A man who weighs 40 percent over his ideal weight at age 45 shortens his life even more: by about 8 months. For women, the risks are substantially lower. Some studies found no loss in life expectancy for women 35 to 45 percent over their ideal weight. Other studies found the risk for overweight women to be about 20 percent lower than the risk for men who were overweight by the same percentage. Moore comments: "The hazards [of obesity] are real – but they are very modest."

Interestingly enough, despite this sex-linked difference, our society is much more tolerant of overweight men than women.

We also know that the cycle of weight loss, followed by regaining weight, losing it again and gaining it back again is much more dangerous to health than maintaining a high but steady weight. And many studies have demonstrated that more than 95 percent of the people who go on weight-loss programs – especially those emphasizing low-calorie diets – will regain all the weight they lose. (Remember Oprah?) In fact, diet companies in the U.S. have been ordered by the government to include a statement on their promotional literature and advertisements explaining that most people who diet to lose weight will eventually gain it back.

More recent research suggests that losing weight may not be as desirable as was once believed. While obesity has been declared a health risk factor, there is no evidence that losing the extra weight actually reduces health risks. In fact, one long-term study of more than 5,000 overweight men and women found that those who lost more than 15 percent of their highest weight were more likely to die younger than those who didn't lose weight. For women, the mortality increased as the amount of lost weight increased.

Other studies of the risks of dieting have found that very low-calorie diets are associated with an increased risk of heart attacks and strokes. (Ironically, the risk of heart attack and stroke is considered to be higher in overweight people, so most people are dieting to reduce these risks!) Dieting is also associated with a lower bone density (the cause of osteoporosis in older women).

One researcher reviewed a large number of studies and concluded: "Dieting is a significant risk factor for obesity." In other words, dieting to lose weight can actually make you fatter.

Many studies have also shown that the location of the extra fat is important. Women are often "pear-shaped," with extra fat on their hips and thighs, but this type of weight distribution is not associated with higher risks. It seems to be riskier to have fat concentrated around the middle.

So what are the medical hazards of obesity? For children, they seem to be fairly minimal. The most significant one is that overweight children tend to become overweight adults, who are at greater risk for some illnesses. Research has found the following increased dangers for overweight children:

- Bone and joint problems. Having to support excess weight can cause knee, hip and foot problems in a developing child.

- Increased risk of breathing problems.

- High blood pressure, which may appear as early as the teen years, and, if it continues into adulthood, can increase the risk of heart attack or stroke.

These risks are not major ones (and they certainly don't justify our strong societal bias against overweight children), but most parents will want to help their overweight child become fitter and closer to an average weight. It is easier to achieve fitness goals in childhood, and if your child adopts healthy eating and exercise habits now, it will not only make him feel better, it may prevent more serious problems in adulthood.

On the other hand, having an overweight child is rarely a reason to panic. Recognize that the health risks are small, and that the risks of low-calorie diets and intensive pressures to lose weight may be much worse.

Is Your Child Overweight?

This should be an easy question to answer, you think. Surely you can tell by looking at the child, or by weighing him or her and comparing that weight to a standard chart. It isn't quite that simple.

Just looking at the child can be terribly misleading. Our ideas about what people of normal weight should look like have been strongly influenced by the fashionable trend towards thinness. One researcher found that the illustrations of girls in school readers have grown progressively thinner over the past 30 years. Marilyn Monroe, who was the "ideal woman" four decades ago, would have to shop in "Plus Size" stores today – she wore a size 16. So when we look at our children (and ourselves), we are often comparing them to an unrealistic and unhealthy standard.

Okay, let's weigh him then and measure his height as well. Unfortunately, that doesn't really tell us much. Recent research has suggested that a much wider range of weights is acceptable at each height than was once believed. Current standards for height and weight are based on a Caucasian population, so any statistics are not helpful for kids who are non-white. We also know that muscle weighs more than fat, so muscular Jimmy may weigh more than his less-athletic friend Bob. But it's really the amount of body fat that is important in determining whether we are fat or fit.

Well then, let's measure body fat. This can also be a challenge. Using calipers (also known as the "skin-fold" test) to measure the thickness of the fat layer on various parts of the body can be informative. (Other methods to measure body fat include submersion in a tank of water – not very practical for home use!) Calculating body fat with this method is probably the best estimate we have, but calipers only measure the external fat, not the internal fat (hidden around the body's internal organs), which is more significant in terms of health and fitness. There is some research to suggest that dieting may reduce only that external and more visible fat but not the internal and more significant fat.

Fine. Let's just go to the doctor. This can be an excellent idea. But remember that your doctor is also part of society and may have some of the same prejudices that the rest of us struggle with. You might prefer to ask for a referral to a doctor with expertise in childhood weight problems, who will be able to assess your child as an individual, not just in comparison to a standard chart.

Concerns about weight are different for children of different ages.

INFANTS

Lesley proudly wheeled her four-month-old daughter Melissa through the mall in her stroller. They were on their way to a doctor's appointment, and Lesley was sure her doctor would be impressed with Melissa's growth and development. Even now, she was bouncing in her stroller seat and smiling at the people they passed.

Then a woman Lesley didn't know approached.

"How old is your baby?" she asked.

"Four months," said Lesley, who was quite used to having people stop and admire Melissa.

"You know, she's really too fat. You should put her on a diet."

"A diet?" Lesley couldn't imagine what this woman was talking about.

"Well, look how fat she is. You should take her off formula and put her on skim milk. And cut back on the pablum."

Lesley was horrified. "But she doesn't have formula or pablum. She's breastfed."

"Well, your milk must be too rich. You should wean her and start her on skim milk."

Fortunately, Lesley went from that encounter to her doctor's office, where she was reassured that her baby was growing well and doing just fine on mother's milk. Not only was weaning her to skim milk unnecessary, it could be very dangerous.

If you've spent any time around babies, you'll probably notice that they grow at different rates and come in a wide variety of sizes. Some seem to be lean and active from birth (and even before birth, as their mothers will tell you); others are quieter, calmer and more likely to gain weight quickly.

How your baby is fed will make a difference, as well. A recent study of growth and development in infants (known as the DAR-LING study) found that breastfed babies often grow very quickly (and can become quite chubby) in the first three or four months. However, after that, breastfed babies usually slow down in their growth rate and are consistently leaner (have a lower percentage of body fat) than formula-fed babies, although they continue to do well developmentally and in terms of overall growth. The researchers found this difference persisted until at least 18 months (the length of the study).

Another study looked at the fat levels of breastfed babies and bottlefed babies in the first weeks of life. While both groups maintained adequate growth and had similar average weights, the bottlefed babies had higher levels of body fat. The breastfed babies gained more muscle and bone density.

This may be one reason why people who were breastfed as infants are less likely to be overweight as adults. There are several possible mechanisms involved here: since a person's fat cells are formed during the first year of life and remain constant after that, the lower number of fat cells created in a breastfed infant's body may mean less tendency to become overweight later on. Another factor may be that breastfed babies regulate their food intake to a much greater extent than bottlefed babies (you can't force a breast-fed baby to keep on nursing when he doesn't want any more, but you can fairly easily get a bottlefed baby to finish the bottle). Or the cause may simply be the different nutritional composition of breastmilk, which may affect the baby's metabolism in ways that we don't yet understand.

The early introduction of solids may also be a factor in exces-sive weight gain in infants. Solid foods should not be introduced before four to six months, and many researchers on this topic feel six months is preferable. When solid foods are begun, the baby should be allowed to take as much or as little as desired – no "just one more spoonful." (We have even seen a parent hold a baby's nose so that he had to open his mouth to breathe – and then another spoonful of cereal was quickly shoved in! When the baby doesn't want any more, he shouldn't be urged or forced to eat any more.) Finger foods are probably the best to begin with, so that the baby really is taking only what his appetite asks for.

Most parents of plump babies find that as the baby becomes more active and graduates from an infant to a toddler, the extra weight disappears. Many babies gain very little weight between 12 and 18 months, for example, as the fat they have is gradually replaced by more muscle.

Even if your baby continues to be chubby, remember that fat is an essential component of the infant's diet (ideally, from breast-milk). There have been cases of babies who were put on skim-milk diets by well-meaning parents who wanted to keep their fat levels down; some of those babies ended up in hospital and some have suffered permanent kidney or brain damage. Babies need fat. It's essential for brain growth and development (which continues through the first three years of life) and because they are growing more rapidly during the first year than at any later stage.

It is valuable, of course, to emphasize the fruits, vegetables and grains that will continue to be an important part of your child's diet as he or she grows. But don't worry about your baby being over-weight or try to cut back on his or her food intake. As long as you are offering healthy foods, the baby's appetite can be your guide.

TODDLERS AND PRESCHOOLERS

Marieke was so frustrated by her son Dieter's lack of appetite that she would do almost anything to get him to eat. He'd been fine as a baby, but now that he was almost two he seemed to eat nothing at all. He was very active and rarely sat still long enough for a meal – two mouthfuls and he'd be asking to "go play" again.

Marieke felt she'd tried everything – making attractive meals, serving small portions, giving him frequent snacks instead of three large meals. Still he didn't seem to eat much.

Her mother-in-law suggested offering him more sweets – cookies, puddings and other dessert-type foods. To Marieke's relief, it worked. Dieter was enthusiastic about the treats and eagerly began eating more of these high-fat, high-calorie foods. Unfortunately, it worked too well, and soon Marieke was beginning to worry about Dieter's weight. He'd gone from a lean and active little boy to a plump one who was less interested in active play.

⚫ It's quite common for toddlers and preschoolers to seem to have little appetite, although parents often worry about it. During the first year of life, the baby grows very rapidly and needs to eat quite a bit in order to accomplish that growth. But the growth rate slows down dramatically after the first year, and the toddler's interest in eating slows down in proportion. This is a normal, self-regulating process and shouldn't be a cause for concern.

It can become a problem, though, when parents respond as Marieke did by giving the child more high-fat foods. Some children love the taste of these foods so much that they will eat more of them than they need – especially if the parents are strongly encouraging them to eat more. This can be the beginning of a weight problem.

Most healthy toddlers and preschoolers will continue to have a rounded look. If they have been breastfed, the muscle development caused by the type of sucking that nursing babies do will give them round "chipmunk" cheeks that can make their faces look fatter. It's also normal for children in this age group to have a rounded and protruding belly – that's not excess fat but simply limited space for a lot of internal organs.

What can be most helpful in preventing obesity or reducing overweight at this age is encouraging the love of activity that is natural in most preschoolers. Avoid using the TV or playpen to keep your child quiet; instead encourage lots of active play, go for walks, climb everything in the playground, play follow-the-leader, play with balls, and so on. It is never too early to make your child's life healthy and active.

THE SCHOOL-AGE CHILD

Weight most often becomes a concern for parents after their child reaches the age of five. Now he may be subjected to teasing by other children, may find it hard to take part in some sports or other school activities or may not be able to wear the same clothes as the other children. He begins to feel different and may start to feel bad about himself.

The activity level of the average child decreases fairly significantly once he or she begins school. Time to play outdoors and run around with friends is cut dramatically; now she's expected to sit quietly at her desk most of the day. She's also more likely to be eating less nutritious foods because she's influenced by television, advertising and friends at school.

Is your child's weight a cause for concern?

The little girl with the stocky build – square shoulders, no waist, solid-looking legs – is probably just fine, even though she doesn't look like a fashion model. And the little boy with a generally rounded build is probably fine, too.

You will be more concerned about a school-aged child whose tummy hangs over the waistband of his pants or who finds his shorts are too tight around his thighs or the girl with visible rolls of fat on her back.

* You can perform your own skin-fold tests without calipers to get a rough idea of the amount of external fat on your child's body. (Ask permission first, of course.) Good places to check for fat may be around the belly-button, the lower back just above the hipbones and the upper arms. You don't have to pinch, just see how much excess fat there is that you can get between your thumb and forefinger. Is there more than an inch? If so, it might be a good time to talk to your child about increasing fitness.

The recommendations and guidelines in this book for eating healthy foods and increasing activity will benefit any child or adult, even if they seem to be of normal weight. They will not encourage rapid weight loss or make a healthy child of stocky build into a thin one, but neither of these goals is desirable anyway.

What if your child is concerned about his or her weight, even though your own observations and perhaps your doctor's assessment convince you that there is no problem? First of all, realize that your child is not unusual. In one study, a majority of fourth grade girls considered themselves overweight and were actively trying to diet to lose weight. Many children as young as five or six are already aware of our societal preoccupation with body size and worry that they aren't thin enough.

You can talk to your child about the information presented in this book, and in particular about the dangers of dieting for children. Let your child know that you accept and love her the way she is. If she wants to become fitter, however, reducing fat in her diet, increasing fiber and increasing exercise will only be beneficial.

3

Why Is My Child Overweight?

Guilt is something all parents suffer from, and parents of over-weight kids often feel that their child's weight is one more thing to feel guilty about. Perhaps friends and relatives – or even the family doctor – have made comments: "How did you let that kid get so fat? Don't you care about his health?"

In response, the parents begin to question themselves. Have they handled mealtimes or feeding problems badly? Have they caused some emotional problem that led to overeating? For parents who place a high value on physical attractiveness, having a chubby child can seem like a failure.

One mother says, "I always felt a bit defensive when I introduced my daughter to people. I'd quickly tell them about how good her grades were in school because I wanted them to see her as more than just this overweight kid. I felt like it reflected on me somehow."

On the other side, it's often easy to fall into anger or resentment about your child's size and blame him or her for being overweight. After all, that's the stereotype: the greedy, lazy, fat person who has no willpower and could be thin if he or she just *tried*. Parents are influ-enced by the high value society places on a slim body just as other people are, and often believe damaging myths about what causes people to be larger than average in size.

The best way to counteract these myths is to consider the research on the real causes of obesity and overweight.

The truth is, we don't really know why some people weigh more than others of the same height and frame. At one time, most of us believed it was a simple equation: take the number of calories consumed (through eating) and subtract the number of calories used up (through exercise). What's left gets stored as fat.

But it isn't so simple, as researchers have discovered. Weight turns out to be a very complex subject. Most of the research on weight and weight loss has been done on adults (primarily women) and only a small percentage of the research looks specifically at children. We can't assume that the results would be the same if children were included in these studies, but some factors seem to be consistent.

Let's look at some of the factors that may be influencing your child's size – and remember that, in most cases, more than one factor will be involved. A recent review of the literature concluded that the following were key factors in weight and body size: heredity (described as the most important factor, responsible for more than 50 percent of the differences in body sizes), eating a high-fat diet (although not necessarily higher in overall calories) and lack of exercise.

Dieting was also identified as a significant factor. Trying to lose weight by controlling calories makes it significantly more likely that the person will be overweight, and the more often the person diets, the higher the probability of becoming overweight. That's one reason why we state so categorically that children should not diet. Restricting food, as diets do, only makes the problem worse.

Let's examine these key factors more closely.

Heredity

When parents Valerie and Tim married, everyone agreed they made an attractive couple. Valerie is small, fine-boned and slender. Tim is a stocky, muscular man who played football in college. As he's gotten older, he's developed a bit of a potbelly.

Today they have four children – two boys and two girls. The boys have inherited their mother's build – they are slender and inclined to be skinny. Valerie remembers: "When Paul was a baby, people were always saying 'What a cute little girl!' just because he was tiny."

The two girls, however, have inherited their dad's body type. Both have round faces and a tendency to be plump. Jennifer says, "I don't think I've ever really had a waist. On my dad, that looks fine, but I keep wishing I looked more like my mom."

Just as a child can inherit Dad's brown eyes and Mom's snub nose, so can he or she inherit a body type that may be inclined to overweight.

Anthropologists and medical researchers use three broad body-type classifications: the ectomorph, the mesomorph and the endomorph. The ectomorph is typically tall and thin (the kind of person who becomes a fashion model). The mesomorph tends to have a more muscular type of body – many athletes (swimmers and track and field stars, for example) would fit into this classification. The endomorph has a rounded type of body with a greater tendency toward plumpness. Think of Mae West as an example.

These body types are consistent throughout the person's lifetime: even though an endomorph may become thin due to illness or an eating disorder such as anorexia, the tendency to a rounder shape is still there. Endomorphs can also become quite muscular and physically fit – many football players fall into this category.

The ectomorph is currently the fashionable standard body type for girls and women while the mesomorph is in style for males. That hasn't always been the case – just look at the plump and voluptuous nudes in the paintings of a few centuries ago. Body types, however, are inherited without regard to gender or fashion. As Valerie and Tim's children have discovered, that can mean having a body that doesn't conform to current styles.

Hereditary factors are those that are in-born and passed from generation to generation through genes – groups of amino acids that are clumped together to form chromosomes. Even the most straightforward hereditary attributes, such as eye color or blood type, are complicated by the fact that our chromosomes come in pairs, with some genes being dominant, squashing the expression of recessive genes. Obesity is much more complicated than blood type. For one thing, with enough energy intake and a minimum of energy expenditure, you can make anyone fat. Also, it is not controlled by just one gene or pair of genes. In fact, the role of genes in obesity is only now becoming clear.

At one time, physicians and researchers played down the role of heredity in the development of obesity. While studies showed that children with two obese parents had an 80 percent chance of becoming obese (compared to a 40 percent chance if one parent was obese or a 3 percent chance if neither parent was obese), experts were quick to suggest that this had more to do with environment than heredity. Children raised by overweight parents, the theory went, would have more high-calorie foods around the house and probably would not be encouraged to be physically active. Kids with obese parents tended to be obese only because they had learned bad eating habits at home.

However, two other studies have suggested that heredity is much more important than was previously believed.

One study looked at the weights of children who had been adopted as infants and compared them to the weights of their biological parents and their adoptive parents. Since the children were raised by the adoptive parents and exposed to the foods and activities enjoyed by the adoptive family, the "learned eating and behavioral habits" theory would suggest that the children would closely match the weights of the adoptive parents. In fact, the results showed that the children's weights were highly correlated with the weights of their *biological* parents and not with the weights of the adoptive parents.

Social workers who organize reunions between birth parents and their children who have been adopted frequently comment on the similarity in body types. They often see a plump child adopted by two slender parents or a slender child in a family with overweight parents – but as soon as the birth parents walk into the room, it's obvious to everyone where the child's body type comes from. (It also often makes it easier for the adoptive parents to relax about their child's weight and stop trying to make him or her match their body type.) American and Danish studies have shown this clearly.

Another study looked at identical twins who were separated at birth and raised by different adoptive families. (Identical twins are ideal for studying heredity because they have the same genetic makeup.) This study found that, as adults, identical twins tended to have very similar weights – usually within a couple of pounds – even though they were raised in completely different families that may have had very different eating habits.

We now have much more direct evidence about hereditary factors in obesity (at least in rats). A number of genes have been identified, starting in 1994, that have a place in controlling weight. The first gene that was discovered was the ob gene, which is responsible for a protein called leptin. It is made in fat tissue and travels through the blood to the brain's satiety center. The more fat in the body, the more leptin and the lower the appetite. In addition, high levels of leptin contribute to the burning of fat. If leptin levels are low, or if a less effective form is made, then obesity can result. The receptor for this protein can also be abnormal, so that even very high levels of leptin do not have an effect. A gene that regulates this receptor has been discovered, as has one (dubbed the "fat" gene) that may both increase appetite and interfere with the processing of fat. Other chemicals involved with appetite control have also been discovered.

⇒> Heredity is a very important factor in obesity and overweight. We can modify our shape to a certain extent by changes in diet and physical activity, but our inherited body type puts limits on the extent of those changes.

Mark and Adam, age 11, were best friends despite being quite different in appearance. Mark's ribs always showed when he wore a bathing suit and his bony knees embarrassed him, but even when he tried to gain weight it didn't seem to make much difference. Adam couldn't understand why he weighed so much more than Mark, because they ate many of the same things and took part in the same activities. They both decided to exercise and change their diets. Mark tried to increase his carbohydrates – eating more bread and potatoes – and began jogging daily. Adam joined him in his daily run and also tried to change his diet to include less fat.

Three months later, after sticking faithfully to their plans, both were definitely fitter. But while Mark had developed more muscle, he was still thin, and Adam was still plump despite having a more muscular physique. While neither of them achieved the goal of the "perfect" body, that doesn't mean their efforts were wasted. Eating well, exercising regularly and becoming fitter are beneficial for children of all shapes and sizes.

In this discussion of heredity it's important to understand how various elements of our physical makeup are inherited. You may be reading this and wondering how the two very heavy parents you know could have produced a slender child, or why three of the children in your family are of normal weight and the fourth is overweight. Remember that two parents, both with brown eyes, can have a child with blue eyes – the blue eyes may be inherited from a generation or two back along the family tree.

Heredity is not a template, passed down from one person to the next, but more like a game of probability. For example, if both parents have brown hair (and there are some genes for blond hair in their family background), the statistics suggest that, of their four children, three will have brown hair and one may have blond hair. However, it is also quite possible for them to have four blond children or even a redhead or two.

Inherited tendencies to body shape and size work the same way. If you are wondering where your heavier-than-average child came from, be sure to look at other branches of your family tree. He may have inherited his size from grandma – just as one of our children, Teresa's son Danny, the only redhead in her family, inherited his hair color from his grandmother.

Overeating

Let's imagine that we spend a day recording the food intake of two ten-year-old girls: Jenny, who is overweight, and Kathy, who is not. We write down the exact amount of every mouthful each girl eats, then calculate the number of calories they have consumed. At the end of the day, who will have taken in more calories?

If you're like most people, you'll pick Jenny. If that was your choice, the results may surprise you. Some researchers performed exactly this experiment, recording the food intake of groups of overweight and normal-weight children, and discovered that, in fact, slender Kathy will probably eat more than her overweight friend.

When Teresa was married, she came up against this seeming paradox on a daily basis. While she was watching her diet carefully, rarely eating desserts other than fruit but still having trouble keeping her weight down, her husband would eat two large bowls of ice cream every night (one after supper and one before he went to bed). And it was the rich, creamy, high-fat brand of ice cream, too. Yet he never gained a pound.

It's also interesting to note that while the percentage of adults in the U.S. who are overweight has increased steadily over the last hundred years, the average food intake has actually decreased over the same period of time. In other words, people are, on average, eating fewer calories (in fact, about 500 calories per day less) than their ancestors did. Despite that, most of them weigh more.

Clearly, the image of the overweight child as someone who eats huge amounts of food doesn't hold up. Why, then, does that image persist? One researcher commented that people tend to notice every bite the overweight person eats (as though they shouldn't be eating anything at all) while they are much less likely to be aware of a thinner person who is snacking or having a second helping of dessert. Overweight children may also eat for comfort or other emotional reasons that make their eating more noticeable.

Researchers have also found that taste preferences – which seem to be in-born – vary quite dramatically from one person to another. In one study, women were offered milkshakes to drink that varied in fat content and the total number of calories. The overweight women consistently chose and preferred the higher-fat drinks, while the more slender women preferred the lower-fat ones – even though the tastes and textures were designed by the experimenters to be very similar. The women in the experiment didn't know which milkshakes were higher in fat and couldn't really say why they chose the ones they did. They just liked them better. Other studies have shown similar results. This is probably related to genetic factors.

Parents often notice that siblings can have very different food preferences. Lenore comes home from school hungry and asks for a salad or a piece of fruit. If she's given a steak or pork chop, she always carefully removes all the fat because she hates the taste of it. Her brother John asks for cookies after school, and if there aren't any he'll make himself a bowl of sugar-sweetened cereal. When Lenore cuts the fat off her meat, John asks if he can eat it. If he has salad, he wants it drowned in a creamy salad dressing. These tastes are not a matter of willpower – Lenore really does prefer salad and fresh fruit, and the taste of fatty meats makes her feel ill – and they aren't easily influenced by parents.

Matthew's parents wanted to discourage him from developing a taste for sweets, so they made sure his first solid foods were vegetables and he didn't get any cookies or treats until he was past two years old. But Matthew's mother still remembers the first time he had ice cream when he was two and a half. "His face just lit up, and he gobbled down that ice cream as though he'd been waiting for it his entire life. And he still has a very sweet tooth – he loves anything with sugar in it."

Fiona's mother was worried about her plump daughter's love of chocolate and candy, so she made sure her school lunches contained only low-calorie, nutritious foods – no cookies, no potato chips, no treats. Then one day Fiona's teacher called. "She told me that Fiona was begging the other kids for their treats and offering to do their homework for a chocolate bar. I realized that restricting her this way not only wasn't fair, but it wasn't working. So I began adding desserts to her lunch," her mother says.

This is where heredity and the environment interact. In a world where chocolate bars and cheezies didn't exist, children like Fiona probably wouldn't be overweight. In fact, her inborn tendency to store fat efficiently and to seek out higher-calorie foods would be a survival factor – if there were a famine, Fiona would outlast many of her skinnier neighbors.

In our present environment, many of us find ourselves in a battle with our bodies. A natural attraction to high-fat foods or a natural tendency to store the calories we get can mean that we end up being overweight.

The Setpoint Theory

Two interesting but related studies looked at weight loss and weight gain in healthy people. In one, a group of normal-weight people were put on a very low-calorie diet for several months. They all lost weight, but became completely obsessed with food – thinking about it constantly, dreaming about it, talking about it. (Anyone who has been on a diet will recognize these symptoms.) As soon as the diet ended, all the subjects quickly returned to their previous weight within a few months. These results are typical and have been repeated in many other studies – most people who lose weight on any kind of diet quickly regain it. One researcher has said, "The faster you lose the weight, the faster you gain it back." Many people, in fact, will gain back more weight and end up fatter than before they started the diet.

Another researcher took a group of prisoners and put them on a very high-calorie diet to make them gain weight (again, all were normal weight to begin with). It's interesting to note that many of them had a great deal of difficulty gaining weight, and had to force themselves to eat large amounts of food and restrict all physical activities. One man, despite eating more than 8,000 calories a day, managed to gain less than ten pounds over several months. Even more interesting, at the end of the study when the prisoners returned to their normal eating patterns, all of them quickly lost the extra weight and ended up very close to their previous weight.

Studies like these have led researchers to develop what is called the setpoint theory. They suggest that each individual body has a weight that it prefers, and that when the person varies from that weight a number of mechanisms come into play to return to that desired weight. Some of us have fairly high setpoints and others have low ones.

What determines our setpoint? We don't know for sure. Certainly, heredity is one factor. Some researchers have suggested that feeding patterns in infancy may be important in creating a setpoint. Babies who are fed infant formula and who start on solid foods early develop a higher setpoint than babies who are breastfed and start solids later. This seems to have more to do with the type of food than the quantity, because in studies where all babies are fed completely on demand, the breastfed babies are still leaner.

A couple of factors are known to change the setpoint. One is dieting. Eating a very low-calorie diet seems to raise the setpoint – as though the body believes it has just survived a famine and intends to increase its fat stores in case it ever happens again. That means the heaviest people are often those who have tried the hardest to lose weight. After repeated dieting, and having to take in fewer and fewer calories at each stage to lose weight, the body's setpoint is pushed up even higher. In adults, this is sometimes described as the yo-yo syndrome, but it happens with children as well.

The only thing that seems to lower the setpoint is regular aerobic exercise – which we mention below but will discuss in more detail in Chapter Five.

Exercise

Richard and Jamie are brothers. They have the same cereal and juice for breakfast, identical lunches (most often a peanut butter sandwich, fruit, carrot sticks and a muffin or potato chips to go with the milk they get at school) and the same foods for supper. Yet Richard is considerably heavier than Jamie.

Let's follow them around for a day. Richard likes to watch TV in the morning while he eats his breakfast and gets ready for school. Jamie, who dreams of being a baseball star, usually gobbles down his cereal and then heads outside to practice batting the ball against the side of the house. At lunch time, Richard generally plays on the swings and slides or talks to his friends; Jamie usually has a basketball game going or plays catch with a friend. After school, Richard usually heads for the TV again. Jamie's more of an outdoor kid who doesn't mind walking several blocks to get to a friend's house for a game of ball or street hockey. (Richard generally asks his mother to drive him where he wants to go.)

These differences are pretty typical. While overweight children often do not eat more than other children, research shows that they are generally much less active. (One researcher wisely points out that it's hard to say which came first: are some children overweight because they are less active, or do they become less active because they are overweight and feel embarrassed about taking part in sports or other activities?)

A few generations ago, physical activity was simply a necessary part of everyone's daily life. Children walked to school (yes, those stories your parents told about walking miles and miles to school may well have been true) and rode horses or bikes to get where they needed to go. Everyone in the family had to help with household chores that typically required a fairly high activity level – cutting the grass, hanging out laundry, etc. Today, many children ride schoolbuses or are driven to school, and definitely expect to be driven almost everywhere else they go. Household chores are kept to a minimum, and transferring wet clothes from the washer to the dryer or cutting the lawn with a ride-on lawnmower doesn't take much exertion.

In our low-exercise society, our bodies – which are designed to be active – are showing the effects. For most people, gaining weight is simply one of the natural consequences of being less active.

One of the chief culprits, especially for children, is television. Children who watch a large amount of TV are not only not out running around and getting exercise, they are actually burning fewer calories than if they were just resting or reading. We will examine the influences of TV and exercise in more detail in later chapters.

Emotional and Psychological Factors

Here it comes, the anxious parent thinks. I knew my child was overweight because of some emotional damage I caused.

You may be reassured to know that research shows overweight children are, in fact, no different emotionally or psychologically than children of average weight. One study found that the range in self-esteem – from high to low – of overweight children was just the same as for the control group of children of normal weight.

Some overweight children do have emotional difficulties, but it is often hard to say which came first: the weight problem or the emotional distress. Since children who don't fit current standards of body size are often teased or ridiculed, it's not surprising that they develop lower self esteem or feel depressed. But it's important to remember that there are also many larger kids who feel self-confident and comfortable about their size.

Reg remembers: "I don't know why my weight didn't bother me much, but it never did. I got teased by kids at school, but many of my relatives have the same build as I do so I felt like I fit in with them."

The support Reg received from his family was probably a very significant factor in his positive feelings about himself. One study found that overweight children with low self-esteem tended to blame themselves for the negative comments made by others. If, during the study, someone teased them about being fat, they responded by saying, "I know I'm too fat, it's my fault, I shouldn't eat so much." These children tended to have low self-esteem and low self-confidence. But another group of overweight children responded to these comments by saying, "It was rude of him to say that. He's got no manners." They disliked the teasing, but put the responsibility on the person saying it. This group tended to have higher self-esteem.

Parents can make a real difference to their child's emotional health by supporting their child's right not to be teased about body size, thus encouraging self-esteem. This is also important because several studies on weight loss and improved fitness have found that self-esteem is a good predictor of success. In other words, those children who feel good about themselves are more likely to become fitter.

Do children eat for comfort? Sometimes. There's no question that food is often very comforting. (Remember the bliss on your baby's face when you nursed her?)

Alice noticed that her ten-year-old son Luke had been gaining weight since she returned to work. When she talked to him, she discovered that he'd been snacking a lot during the hour and a half between the time he got home from school and the time she got home from work. "How do you feel when you're here on your own?" she asked, and he admitted that he was lonely and missed her.

Together they were able to work out some solutions: he could invite a friend to come over to the house with him, he could call Alice at work if he's feeling lonely and Alice would prepare some snacks specifically for that after-school time. She chose foods that would appeal to him without being too high in fat and calories, and tucked in some notes that said "I love you" and "I'm thinking about you" and "I really liked that painting you did last week."

If you think that eating for comfort may be a factor in your child's weight gain, be sure you find other ways to meet those needs. Providing as much physical contact as possible may be helpful – can you have a morning snuggle together in bed? A cuddle-up story-reading time? Even quick hugs and pats on the back can make a difference. Don't expect your child to simply cut back on comfort foods once his behavior has been pointed out to him. That need for comfort is real, and he needs your help in meeting it.

Parents also sometimes unintentionally teach their children to use food to suppress strong emotions. It's easy when your two-year-old is having a violent temper tantrum to offer a cookie or other treat as a distraction. It often works, too.

Aleisha remembers: "I had no idea children could be so emotional until Amy hit two. She'd have tantrums over nothing, and sometimes it really scared me. I was relieved to discover that she'd stop screaming if I gave her something she liked, a cookie, an ice cream cone, a candy." After a while, though, Aleisha realized that she was relying on these treats to cope with Amy's emotional states. "If she was mad at me, if she was unhappy or disappointed about something, if she was scared – food always seemed to work."

But she wasn't motivated to make a change until she noticed that Amy, now four and a half, was beginning to use food the same way. If she got upset about something, she'd head for the fridge. Aleisha could see this as the beginning of a lifelong approach to dealing with emotions.

While the role of emotional and psychological factors in weight gain is not entirely clear (by the same token, we don't really understand the emotional causes of anorexia, either), it is very clear that overweight children need plenty of emotional support. You can help your child to feel good about herself and have high self-esteem even if she is larger than average. Trying to convince her to lose weight by shaming or criticizing her will only make things worse.

Body Changes and Puberty

Children do not grow steadily and evenly, despite the appearance of that nice smooth line on the growth charts. You may remember that when your child was a baby, he or she went through growth spurts – times of eating voraciously and growing rapidly. These were often followed by a plateau period when the baby's rate of growth (and appetite) decreased again.

School-age children continue this growth pattern, although it is less obvious (probably because we weigh them less often) – with one exception. As children approach puberty (and the age at which puberty begins can vary quite dramatically – it can start as young as eight for some girls), they often go through a period of weight gain just before their growth spurt begins. This can be difficult because it's often happening at an age when the child is becoming quite self-conscious and aware of his or her appearance.

Danny had always been quite a skinny child whose ribs showed no matter how much food he ate. But after he turned 12, he began to put on weight, and by the beginning of summer he had a noticeable roll of fat around his tummy. That summer, though, he grew four inches and by fall had regained his leaner physique.

Girls approaching puberty must have a certain percentage of fat in their bodies in order to begin menstruation. (Anorexic girls will delay the onset of menstruation or, if they have already begun having periods, will stop menstruating until their body fat levels rise again.) Their entire shape changes as hips and breasts develop. It's very common for a child at the beginning of this stage to look quite chubby, but it's a normal – and essential – part of the body's preparation for the maturing process.

"I remember Lindsey being in despair because her Aunt Judy told her she was getting fat. Well, she was definitely plumper than she had been a year before. I didn't know what to do about it," recalls Cindy.

She finally took Lindsey to their family doctor, who pointed out the early signs of puberty "That was two years ago," Cindy says. "About a year ago, she shot up and grew about five inches, developed breasts and started her period – and now I can hardly believe she was once so chubby."

If you have noticed a sudden increase in appetite and a corresponding weight gain in your pre-adolescent, consider that it may be a sign of approaching puberty. Has the weight gain been accompanied by the development of pubic hair or underarm hair? In girls, you may notice the growth of breast buds; boys may find their testicles beginning to grow. If these other signs are present, the weight gain is probably just a preparation for the growth spurt that marks puberty.

Medications and Medical Conditions

There are some medical conditions, both inherited and acquired, that include overweight or obesity as a symptom, but these conditions all have other symptoms as well. For example, thyroid problems that cause children to be overweight also cause them to be unusually short or to stop growing. If you have any concerns about your child's health, it is essential to have him or her checked out by a physician.

Some medications, particularly steroids, can also cause weight gain.

"My niece Zoe was quite a slender baby," says Anne. "Then she had a couple of seizures and the doctor decided she needed to be on medication to prevent more seizures. I heard all this over the phone, but I didn't see Zoe for a couple of months. When I did, I was shocked. She was so fat you could hardly see her eyes, she just had this completely round face and her arms and legs looked like sausages." As Zoe grew older, however, her doctor was able to adjust the medication and her weight came down again.

If you are concerned that a particular medication your child must take is causing weight gain, it's also important to discuss this with your doctor.

Why Is My Child Overweight?

To summarize, there are no absolute or definite causes. In fact, it's easier to explain what the causes of overweight are *not*:

- Your child is not overweight because you are a bad parent.
- Your child is not overweight because he is lazy, greedy, weak, stupid or lacking in willpower.

For all the attention that is paid to body size and weight in our society, we still have very little solid information on the causes of excess weight and obesity. The causes are probably different for each person and it remains a complex condition, but it is important to realize that no one is at fault here, neither you nor your child.

4

❧

Teasing and Self-Esteem

Tony joins his friends at lunch time in the schoolyard. It's a cold winter's day, and the shallow creek that runs across the back of the school property has frozen solid. The boys decide to go sliding and head for the ice.

Tony watches the others for a minute or two, then scrambles down the gently sloping bank and onto the ice. Right away one of the other boys starts to shout, "Look out, Tony's on the ice! It's cracking already!" Others join in: "You're too fat, Tony, you'll break right through!"

He knows they're "only teasing," but it hurts. Tony feels his face turn red and it isn't just from the cold wind. He tries to ignore them and join in the sliding games, but his stomach hurts and he isn't having much fun.

Anja is invited to a sleepover party at her friend Ruby's, and she's pretty excited about going. But when she gets there, the girls spend most of the time discussing their appearances and boys. Two of them start whispering together and looking at Anja. Finally one giggles and says, "Say, Anja, your stomach's getting pretty fat. Are you sure you're not pregnant?"

Another girl laughs and says, "No, she's always been fat."

"Fatty, fatty, two-by-four, can't get through the kitchen door!" chants another.

Anja struggles not to cry in front of the other kids. She wants to phone her mother to come and get her, but she's afraid they'll laugh at her even more. So she endures a night of teasing ("Where did your mother buy you this nightgown, Anja – in the maternity department?") and cries herself to sleep as quietly as she can.

Being overweight may not be a significant risk to your child's physical health, but it can certainly damage children's self-esteem if they're subjected to the kinds of teasing most large-sized children encounter.

Why do children tease their heavier friends and classmates? For one thing, it's socially acceptable. While children would be condemned by most adults for making racist remarks or making fun of a disabled child's handicap, they can't help but be aware of our society's bias against overweight people of all ages. They may have heard their parents make fun of an overweight relative, they may have heard "fat jokes" on television, they may have read books (including *Blubber* and others, by popular author Judy Blume) in which the heavy child is seen as a ridiculous figure who can be teased and humiliated freely by the book's heroes.

It isn't just classmates and friends who can be cruel in these ways. Siblings often tease their heavier brothers or sisters about their size without fear of being rebuked by their parents. In fact, the parents sometimes secretly hope the teasing will shame or encourage their child to lose weight. Instead of stopping the other children's hurtful comments, they might tell the overweight child, "You know, if you just lost some weight the other kids would stop teasing you."

Why do we permit this kind of teasing and cruelty when we'd be quick to put a stop to racist comments or other insensitive behavior? In part, it's because we still subscribe to some of the myths about being overweight that we discussed in previous chapters. We believe (perhaps subconsciously, because we have heard this message for so many years) that the overweight person should lose weight for his or her own good, and that he or she could lose weight with just a little effort. It isn't like having a physical disability or belonging to a minority culture, something that a person can't help or do anything about. Because we are still affected by our society's biases, we allow children to express those biases, often in very hurtful ways.

Of course, you can't educate everyone your child may meet, and so teasing and unkind comments will continue to be a problem. What you can do is provide your child with concrete strategies to deflect teasing.

How to Counteract Teasing

If the Teasing Happens in Your Presence, Be Firm about Stopping It

As an adult, you need to make it very clear that this kind of behavior is unacceptable. Be firm and straightforward about your feelings with the child who has made the comment, and don't permit it to continue.

This can be particularly difficult if you are overweight yourself, because you might be afraid that the child will insult you, too. And just like children, adults hate having their size commented on. But it's very important to let the child know that this kind of teasing is wrong. Your reaction will also mean a lot to the child who is being teased – when you ignore the comments, your child may suspect or believe that you agree with them. He needs your support.

At Jennifer's birthday party, the meal was being served buffet-style. Because she was the birthday girl, her mother let her go through the line first. Melina, one of the party guests, commented in a loud voice, "Oh, great, once Fatty goes through the line there won't be any food for the rest of us." Jennifer's mother could see how hurt her daughter was. She put her hand on Melina's shoulder and said, "If you're worried about not getting enough to eat, I promise that there will be plenty of food for everyone. But I didn't like the way you called Jennifer 'Fatty.' That's a hurtful name and it's not very polite to comment on people's bodies." Melina didn't say anything, but she looked a bit embarrassed. Jennifer had been apprehensive when her mother started talking, but she looked relieved when she saw Melina's reaction.

There are many possible ways to handle teasing situations. Stay calm and try some of the following:

"I think that hurt Bobby's feelings, and I don't want you to say things like that any more."

"We don't make fun of the way people look."

"People come in all shapes and sizes, and it isn't polite to tease people about their size."

"I understand that you're upset with your sister, but you need to discuss the problem with her, not tease her. You're just trying to hurt her feelings, and I won't allow you to do that. Now let's talk about the problem."

Remember, no one has the right to criticize another person's body or appearance in a hurtful way. Just because a child is overweight doesn't mean he deserves to be teased. He doesn't, and he needs you to defend him.

Be an Advocate for Your Child

Recent research on bullying shows that contrary to popular thinking, bullying can be significantly reduced if you report it to the school and the school takes action. Principals and teachers may need to be pushed to take an antibullying stance, and some cannot be convinced to do so. Most bullying takes place where teachers can't see it, so don't be surprised if school officials tell you they don't have a bullying problem.

If You Only Hear about the Teasing Afterward, Encourage Your Child to Express His or Her Feelings

Again, our society's bias against larger-size people puts children at a real disadvantage when they are teased about their weight. A black child faced with racist insults can at least find understanding and acceptance within his own family. But the overweight child who comes home from school upset and tearful because of the teasing he's been through is often greeted by the same attitude at home: "Well, why don't you lose some weight then?"

That isn't what your child needs. He needs your support and empathy to cope with what can be a very painful experience.

Listen to Steven talking to his Dad:

Steven: "I hate swimming."

Dad: "You do? You used to love swimming. Did something happen today at swimming class?"

Steven: "Well, sort of."

Dad: "You sound sad about something." (Dad is trying to identify how Steven is feeling.)

Steven: "Some of the kids were teasing me about being fat."

Dad: "How did that make you feel?"

Steven: "Bad. Really bad. They call me Chubbo. And when it was my turn to dive they all made fun of me and said stuff like tidal wave coming."

Dad: "And then how did you feel?"

Steven "Awful. I didn't even want to do my dive."

Dad: "You felt so bad you didn't want to dive." (Here Dad is using what is called "reflective listening" – he's letting Steven know he understands what he's trying to say by reflecting the message back to him. This can be a good way of making sure your child knows he or she is being heard correctly.)

Steven: "But I did. And you know what? The coach said I did the best dive out of the whole class!" (He smiles.)

Dad: "You seem pretty pleased about that."

Steven: "Yeah. I really do like swimming. But I really hate being teased."

Dad: "It hurts when the other kids tease you." (Dad is trying hard to keep from offering suggestions. Once you start telling the child what to do, you cut off the flow of feelings and information.)

Steven: "I get teased in school, too." (He stares at the floor, sadly.)

Dad: "That really bugs you."

Steven: "Yes, it does. I don't know why some kids are so mean." (Long pause.) "I think I'm just going to tell them to stop it. And if they don't, I won't play with them any more. Because, you know, the kids I really like, like Daniel and Nilesh, never tease me."

Dad: "That sounds like a good idea. And you know, I'd like to see you do that new dive. Maybe we could go to the pool this weekend and you could show me?"

That conversation wasn't easy for Dad. He felt a lot of different emotions: anger at the children who were teasing his son, embarrassment that his son was overweight and not the muscular athlete he had hoped for, pride at Steven's successful dive and concern about Steven's feelings and self-esteem. But he realized that it was more important, at that time, for Steven to talk about how he felt and to come up with his own plan for dealing with the teasing.

How can you help your child express feelings? Although some kids will resist talking about their feelings no matter what you say, here are some helpful techniques to try to get them talking about how they feel:

Reflective listening. Dad demonstrated this several times in the conversation with Steven. Reflective listening means rephrasing the child's statements to describe what you think he is feeling. You might interpret facial expressions or body language as well to give you clues about what emotions the child is experiencing, and then tell him or her your impressions.

If you've guessed wrong (for example, if you say, "You seem sad that your friend said that to you" and your child responds, "No, I was really mad!") that's okay. The whole purpose of reflective listening is to let the child know you are paying attention and to discover whether or not you are getting the message accurately. Letting him correct you is one way of helping him to express his feelings more clearly.

Young children sometimes don't have the vocabulary to describe their feelings and might not be able to tell you how they feel. It can be very helpful to use this reflective listening to give them names for their emotions. When they talk about wanting to hurt someone, or even if they can't do more than pound on the floor with their fists, you can describe that emotion for them: "Boy, are you ever angry!" Being able to describe emotions with words helps us deal with them without having to act them out.

Use "um," "uh-huh," "and then what?" These little noises or phrases are ways of encouraging your child to keep talking without you commenting on or judging what she's said. Say it in a friendly, open tone of voice and your child will often continue talking in a more expressive way.

Here's a conversation between Lileth and her mother:

Lileth: "I'm never going back to school."

Mother: "Oh?"

Lileth: "Never. As long as I live. I hate that school. And I hate every single kid in it."

Mother: "Uh-huh?"

Lileth: "You won't believe what happened. I was wearing my new red skirt and Morgan came up to me and said that anyone as fat as me should never wear red."

Mother: "And then what happened?"

Lileth: "Well Julie Simpson was with her and she started laughing and I was so embarrassed I thought I would die. I wished I would die!"

Mother: "Uh-huh." (She nods her head sympathetically.)

Lileth: "Anyway, then the teacher came down the hall and we had to go to class so she couldn't say anything else. But I was really upset all through class. Really upset."

Mother: "I bet."

Lileth: "But you know what? I like red. I don't care what Morgan and Julie think, I'm gonna keep wearing red."

Lileth is clearly an expressive child who talks readily about her feelings. But if her mother had reacted to her first statement – "I'm never going back to school" – by saying what she was thinking ("You can't drop out of school, you're only 12 years old!"), the conversation would have ended right there. Instead, her noncommittal remarks and encouraging noises helped Lileth to tell her mother the underlying story and to find her own solution.

If your child is less expressive, these quietly encouraging comments may need to be accompanied by a lot of patience. Be prepared to have some long periods of silence as your child struggles to deal with some strong emotions, and don't rush to fill in the silence with your own guesses or judgments. Being patient lets your child know that her feelings are important to you and that you're willing to take as long as necessary to let her figure out a way to tell you about them.

Don't judge or criticize feelings. It can be hard for a child to identify or express feelings. If you are critical or negative about those feelings, it will be twice as hard for your child to express them next time.

As children, many of us learned that some of our feelings were unacceptable, and we tend to pass that message on to our children. But in fact, all feelings or emotions are neutral – they aren't good or bad, they just are.

Here's Sabra reacting to her older brother's teasing:

Sabra: "I hate Eli. I wish he was dead."

Mother: (Her first reaction is to tell Sabra that she doesn't hate Eli, that he's her brother and she shouldn't hate him, and that it's terrible to wish somebody dead. But she manages to hear the emotion behind that angry statement.) "Sounds like Eli did something to make you mad."

Sabra: "He said I was fat and lazy and I'll never learn to ride a bike because I'm so fat. He's such a jerk. I really, really hate him."

Mother: (again looking for the feelings behind the words) "You're really mad at Eli. He insulted you and hurt your feelings."

Sabra: (starting to cry) "I hate being so fat. Maybe Eli's right. Maybe I'll never learn to ride a bike."

Mother: "It can be hard to learn to ride a bike – I think it took me about a month before I could do it. I can come and help you after I finish this brief I'm working on."

Sometimes children's emotions are very intense. They haven't learned, as adults have, to hide them or tone them down. But allowing them to express those feelings without judgment or condemnation helps them accept themselves and boosts their self-esteem. (Actions, of course, are a different matter. If Sabra had acted on her feeling of wanting Eli to be dead, by trying to strangle or hit him, her mother would naturally have to intervene. But the words were just Sabra's way of expressing her very strong emotions.)

Anger, the emotion we tend to be most concerned about when it is expressed by children, is often a secondary emotion. The child first feels hurt, disappointed, afraid, or some other emotion, and then quickly becomes angry at the person or other cause of that negative feeling. While a constantly angry child can be a problem, to be able to feel and express anger is actually very healthy. It's much better for Sabra to be angry at Eli for insulting her than for her to accept his hurtful comments and begin to believe them. Anger can be an expression of healthy self-esteem; the child who never seems angry, even when someone else has treated him or her badly, may be accepting the mistreatment because of low self-esteem.

Try not to respond to emotional outbursts with "You shouldn't feel that way." Allow your child to experience and accept the emotions that are there – then you can begin dealing with the causes.

Share your own experiences and feelings. Self-disclosure is one of the most important ways of achieving closeness between two people. If parents can share their own doubts, negative experiences and emotions, it is much easier for their child to do the same.

Leif talks to his daughter Astrid:

Leif: "Mom said you were teased in school today."
Astrid: "I don't want to talk about it." (She stares at the floor, but stays close to her dad. That makes him suspect that she's willing to continue the conversation and might be persuaded to open up a bit more.)

Leif: "That's okay." (He pauses.) "You know, I used to get teased quite a bit when I was a kid."

Astrid: "Oh sure."

Leif: "I did. See this tummy? Well, I was pretty chubby when I was a kid, too. And I wore braces."

Astrid: "Braces?"

Leif: "Yeah, to straighten my teeth. So half of the kids made fun of me for being overweight and the other half made fun of me for being a metalmouth. It was awful."

Astrid: (in a joking tone of voice) "Aw, poor daddy."

Leif: "Yeah, I really hated being teased."

Astrid: "Me too. You know, I thought Alyssa was my friend. I really did. And then she said all these things to me today. I couldn't believe she would do that. How can someone be your friend and then make fun of you for being fat?"

At the beginning of the conversation, Leif didn't know what had happened to Astrid, so he couldn't really talk about her feelings. But sharing his own story let her know that he would understand her experience.

You don't have to have been an overweight child to have a story to share with your child. All children are teased about something: wearing glasses, wearing braces, having funny clothes, having weird parents, doing badly in school, doing well in school, doing badly at sports, and so on. In fact, sharing stories about being teased for reasons other than body size can be very helpful to your overweight child – it lets her know that teasing is a part of life for most children. Maybe that knowledge will help her feel less personally attacked by the cruel words.

Of course, teasing about weight is more painful and more powerful than most other kinds of teasing because it feeds into society's overall prejudice against larger-size people.

Strategies for Coping with Teasing

Most of the time, teasing happens at school, in the playground or in other situations where you can't be there to intervene. Often teachers ignore or are unaware of these situations as well. Regardless of whether adults are present, children need help in developing strategies to deal with the hurtful comments they hear.

Children without these coping strategies may begin to believe some of the hurtful comments they hear. Even with support and encouragement from parents at home, their self-esteem can be damaged and they may begin to see themselves as victims who deserve to be insulted. With some techniques to combat teasing, your child can feel empowered and competent even in the face of negative remarks.

Some techniques to try:

Brainstorm with Your Child

Once she has told you about a teasing situation, ask her how she would like to handle the situation if it happens again. Take some time to discuss possibilities and make a written list of ideas. Don't comment on or evaluate the ideas as she suggests them; just write them down. In fact, it can help if you throw in a few outrageously silly ideas that will help her be more creative.

Here's a list of possible solutions that Sam came up with after being teased by some of the boys on his hockey team:

1. Take all the boys into the change room and beat them up.
2. Have Dad take all the boys out of the arena and beat them up. Maybe I'll help him.
3. Quit hockey.
4. Transfer to another team.
5. Never pass the puck to Jules or Ivan again.
6. Tell Jules he's a pizza-face because he's got bad zits.

7. Move to another city.
8. Ignore them and just keep on playing.
9. Tell the coach about them.
10. Tell them to shut up.

After the list was completed, Sam and his dad looked it over. They eliminated a few as being impractical (such as moving to another city) and others were simply vetoed by his dad as inappropriate (beating the boys up). Sam decided he liked hockey too much to quit and he didn't want to insult Jules because he already knew how much those comments could hurt. So he finally picked solution number 10: he'd tell Jules and Ivan to shut up if they teased him again. His backup plan was to ignore them and keep on playing. Frankly, his parents were skeptical, but to everyone's surprise, except Sam's, it worked. The other boys stopped making comments and the whole team played better.

Help Your Child to Understand Why Kids Tease

Some kids who are continually insulting and mean to others are reacting to stresses in their own lives. Perhaps they have been teased by parents or relatives at home and see it as a normal way of relating to other people. Often it's because knocking other people down seems to be a way of building themselves up.

Sarah's life was being made miserable by one of her classmates, Marci, who continually teased her about her weight and told her she was ugly. Sarah's father made a point of talking to Marci's parents one day at a school open house and discovered that both of them were very concerned about weight and appearance. In fact, they commented that they were "very strict about Marci's diet" and were worried that Marci might be "a little" overweight.

Once Sarah's father had shared that experience with his daughter, Sarah could understand the reasons behind Marci's teasing. She still didn't like it, but she stopped taking it so personally. She even told her parents that she felt sorry for Marci: "It must be awful to have to live that way, always feeling like you don't look good enough, worrying about every single bite you eat. No wonder she says those things to me."

It isn't always possible for parents to meet the children who are teasing their own. But you can encourage your children to consider these questions when they are teased:

- Does he seem unhappy about something (and he's taking it out on you)?

- Has somebody been teasing him (and so now he's teasing you)?

- Is he mean to other children too (so his comments about you are obviously just part of a larger pattern and shouldn't be taken too personally)?

Remind them that children who feel secure in themselves don't need to tease others. These insults are an attempt to make those children feel better. It's important for children to understand the motivations behind teasing so that they don't see it as their fault, something they deserve because they are overweight. No one deserves to be teased, insulted or made fun of for any reason.

Ignoring Teasing Often Works Well

Lucas was having a real problem with some of the kids at school. They'd tease him about his size and he'd explode, telling them to shut up and threatening to beat them up if they said one more word. That just seemed to encourage them to say even more insulting things and Lucas would become even more upset. Finally, his teacher invited Lucas and his mother to a meeting and made a suggestion: that Lucas simply try ignoring the teasing.

It was pretty tough for Lucas to do. When Pierre came by during gym class and said, "You'll never make it around the track, Fatty," he felt his face turn red. But he just kept going and didn't respond. Pierre was surprised that he hadn't elicited the usual reaction, so he went a step further: "Hey, Fatty, I can see your boobs bouncing."

Lucas gritted his teeth and continued. Pierre made a couple more comments, but it soon got boring when Lucas continued to ignore him. After a while, Pierre stopped trying to bother Lucas and joined in some other activities instead.

It took some time for the teasing to decrease significantly. At first, the other children reacted to Lucas's new strategy by teasing him more than they had before. But Lucas had been prepared for that possibility by his teacher, and he continued to control himself and not respond.

As time went by, ignoring the other children began to work. Teasing isn't much fun if you don't get a reaction. The kids who had been teasing Lucas eventually found someone else to tease and stopped bothering him. Lucas also felt better about himself when he learned that he could control his reactions and not let other people upset him.

You may have to help your child learn how to ignore teasing. Some volatile children find this very difficult. Some possible strategies include:

- **Count to ten (or a hundred, or whatever is necessary).** Teach your child to count silently to herself instead of reacting. Tell her to keep counting until the teasing comments have stopped or until she feels calm enough to go on with what she was doing.

- **Walk away.** This isn't always possible, of course, especially if the teasing takes place in class. But if your child is in the playground or some other open setting, he might just quietly walk away when the teasing is bothering him. It isn't any fun to tease somebody who isn't there!

- **Change the topic or continue talking as though you didn't hear the teasing comment.** If the conversation has been focusing on body size and the comments are getting quite insulting, your child could try ignoring them and changing the topic: "Did you see that TV show last night?" or "When did Mrs. Robinson say we were having a math test?" If her conversation has been interrupted by an insult, she could try to continue talking as though the words were never said. She may be aware of her face flushing, but this is rarely as noticeable to others as it is to the person experiencing it.

- **Do something physical.** Controlling your response to teasing can be hard, and some kind of physical action can help. Lucas was running around the track when Pierre started to tease him and it helped him to be able to keep running. In a classroom or other indoor situation, it might help to quietly tap fingers together or to tighten and relax certain muscles.

- **Breathe slowly and deeply.** When we feel upset or tense, we tend to take short, shallow breaths. Deliberately slowing down our breathing can help us relax, and concentrating on taking slow, deep breaths changes our focus. Show your child how to do relaxing breathing at home and encourage him to use it when he's teased elsewhere.

Ignoring teasing can be a surprisingly powerful approach, but it takes a lot of self-control that your child may need time and practice to achieve. Be patient and understanding; make sure he doesn't feel like he's failed if he blows it and gets upset when he's teased.

Teasing Can Sometimes Be Deflected by Humor

In a sense, using humor is a way of ignoring the teasing. Not every child can use humor effectively – it requires quick thinking and the right kind of mind (how many of us think of great snappy comebacks an hour or so after the incident has happened?). There's also a danger of the child overusing self-deprecating humor to the point where it damages his self-esteem – some children seem to insult themselves first before anyone else gets a chance. The other kids may laugh, but the child is still in pain – and he's hurting himself.

Humor works best when it's spontaneous and not hurtful to anyone, including the child making the joke.

Telling the Others to Stop Can Work Well

Bobby's friend Emily had started calling him "Bobby Blubber" every time she saw him. He hated it, but she seemed to think it was funny. Ignoring it didn't seem to make a difference either. He really liked playing with Emily, except for these teasing comments, and didn't know what to do.

Bobby's mother suggested that he let Emily know how he felt and ask her to stop.

Bobby was horrified. "She'll tell me I'm a suck and she'll keep on doing it and she'll probably never want to play with me again."

"I don't think that'll happen, Bobby. But what's the alternative? What if you don't tell her and things go on the same way? You're not very happy about your friendship right now."

Bobby thought for a moment. "I guess you're right. I really want her to stop."

When Emily came over the next afternoon, he decided to risk everything. "Em," he said nervously, "I really hate it when you call me Bobby Blubber and I want you to stop."

"Oh, come on," Emily said. "It's just a nickname."

"Well, I don't like it and I want you to stop."

"Well, if it bothers you that much…"

"Yeah, it does."

"Okay, okay, I won't say it any more. Now can we get out the Lego?"

Because Emily and Bobby were good friends and she valued the friendship, she was quite willing to stop the teasing once she understood that it upset him.

It isn't always that easy. Die-hard teasers and those who are putting down other children in order to build up their own self-esteem are less likely to stop just because they've been asked. However, just having said it can sometimes help the overweight child feel better about himself or herself. It takes some courage and strength to tell other children to stop teasing, and your child may feel pride in having been able to do it, even if the teasing doesn't end. In the end, how your child feels about himself is the most important result.

Building Self-Esteem at Home

You may not be able to prevent or stop all the teasing that goes on in the outside world, but you can make your home a safe haven for your child, a place where she knows she will be accepted, loved and never teased about her size (or anything else, for that matter). In fact, she should be given extra support and reassurance that she is loved and lovable to help compensate for the discouraging comments she may hear elsewhere.

How can you give this support?

Deal with Your Own Feelings
about Being the Parent of an Overweight Child

You may have believed some of the myths about overweight children being lazy or greedy that research has disproved. You might have struggled with a weight problem since childhood yourself, and may be transferring all the negative comments you've heard to your child.

Educating yourself about body size is probably the best step you can take to help you feel more positive about your own body as well as your child's.

"I experienced a real revelation when we were taking photos at Christmas time," Reva says. "I always refused to be in any photos because I was too fat. I even threw away photos of me that other people brought over. Then Shoshie said she didn't want to be in the pictures either, because she was fat. I kept telling her she wasn't fat, but I realized that she was just doing what I had always done. What a terrible message I'd been giving her!"

Reva knew she had to make some changes, for her own sake as well as Shoshie's. She decided to go for counseling to improve her self-esteem.

Not all parents need counseling, of course, but it's important to be aware of feelings about body size that we may be carrying around from our own past experiences and that may be based on false ideas.

Have a Family Policy against Teasing

Some parents think that teasing children frequently at home will help to toughen them up and prepare them for being teased in the outside world. The theory is that if they're used to teasing and insults at home (all done in fun, of course), they won't be upset if they get teased at school or in the playground.

Research, however, has shown that the opposite is true. Children who are teased at home are more distressed by teasing at school, tend to make more hurtful comments to other children and have lower self-esteem.

Children can respond best to a stressful outside environment when they feel securely loved at home. It's important to include siblings in this family policy as well as parents, because brothers and sisters can sometimes be the most insulting of all. Make it as clear as possible that you won't allow people in the family to make fun of each other, to hurt other people's feelings or to tease or call names. It may not be possible to eliminate teasing altogether – sibling rivalry is a reality – but you can focus on treating each other with respect.

When you hear a hurtful comment, simply offer a reminder: "We don't say things like that in our family. That could hurt someone's feelings."

Give Lots of Physical Affection

All of us need physical affection, and for babies and young children it's one of the primary ways that they experience the feeling of being loved.

It's even more important, though, for the overweight child who may feel that his body is disgusting, unattractive and untouchable. These feelings are very damaging to the child's sense of self-worth.

How can you increase physical affection? It's easy once you become aware of it. Some children are naturally more cuddly than others and will enthusiastically respond to any encouragement you give them to sit on your lap, cuddle up at story time or give hugs and kisses. Others are more restrained, and for these children you might find that a casual arm around the shoulders, a pat on the back or a quick hug will work better.

Elise realized that she was giving her eight-year-old daughter Shannon very little physical affection. "I have to confess that it was at least partly because she was overweight," she says. "I didn't like touching those rolls of fat and that big stomach. So when she came for a hug or something, I'd just kind of squeeze her shoulders."

But Elise noticed Shannon becoming more withdrawn and not asking for hugs as often, and she decided her attitude had to change. "She needed my love, overweight or not," Elise says. "I began deliberately giving her long hugs and making myself be aware of her body. Yes, it was fat. And you know what? It wasn't so bad. Pretty soon, it didn't bother me at all. I started reading books to her and she'd cuddle up beside me on the couch, and we both really enjoyed it. And we hug a lot."

Elise found that once she made the effort, she could accept and feel comfortable with Shannon's body even though she was overweight.

Cuddling with Shannon was easy because she was a child who openly asked for physical affection. For Tom and his son Gary, it was more difficult. "Gary wasn't very cuddly, even as a baby," Tom says. "And by the time he was nine, we rarely touched at all. I have to admit that I'm the same way. But I also could see that he needed some expression of love from me to help him feel better about himself."

Hugs and kisses were out of the question. Tom tried a different approach – he offered to give Gary massages. "He was tense from school anyway, and I told him this would help get rid of his headaches. It did, but even more than that, it helped us to feel closer."

It was a big step for Gary to be able to take his shirt off and have his father rub his back, but it benefited both of them. Tom also makes a point of patting Gary on the back, squeezing his hand and sitting close to him whenever possible.

The idea is to let your children know they are loved in the most basic way – through physical demonstrations of affection. It also helps them feel more positively about their bodies, even if they are overweight. If you can hug them in a loving way, their bodies must be okay.

Look for Positive Things to Say about Your Child

We all have more aspects to ourselves than just body size. Unfortunately, it's common for the life of an overweight child to become completely focused on food or weight. She's praised if she loses weight, condemned if she gains it or stays the same; she's criticized for eating and praised for skipping a meal or dessert. Other accomplishments may be ignored, as if they are unimportant compared to weight.

That perspective couldn't be more wrong. It's much more helpful to focus on your child's good qualities and achievements and to recognize that body size is a minor aspect of his or her life.

Some ideas:

- **Avoid labels.** In many families, one child is identified as the smart one, another as the pretty one, another as the athletic one. Your overweight child may already have picked up a label as the fat one. These labels are damaging and limiting to both the child and his or her siblings. (One woman, who grew up in a family where she was the pretty one and her older sister was the smart one, was nearly 30 years old before she realized that these labels were not mutually exclusive and that she was not only pretty but smart as well. Although she had dropped out of high school when she was younger, she has returned to university and is now getting straight A's.) You may have to work hard to discourage relatives from sticking labels – even seemingly positive ones – on your child. If Aunt Mary says, "Oh yes, Jenny's fat but she's the smart one, isn't she?" you can respond with something like, "Yes, Jenny does do well in school and we're also excited that she's started gymnastics this fall. Would you like to see her somersault?" Children need to know that they have many areas in which they can succeed and that they are capable of many accomplishments.

- **Try a self-esteem game for the whole family.** One way of playing this is to have one family member sit in a chair. Then the rest of the family take turns saying positive things about that person. After everyone has had a turn, the person in the chair joins the others in the circle and someone else has a turn in the chair. While this can be embarrassing at first, it ends up boosting the person's self-esteem considerably. Similar games can be played with written lists or other ways of conveying these positive messages.

- **Help your child keep a journal, emphasizing her daily accomplishments.** For this, you will need to plan about 15 minutes of time each evening to help your child to write (or, for younger children, to dictate while you write) her recollections of that day. Ask questions such as "What did you enjoy doing the most?" and express your own pleasure and pride in her achievements. This will give her a private record of positive experiences that she can refer to whenever she likes.

- **Deliberately look for things to praise or comment on in an encouraging way.** It doesn't have to be anything big: "Thanks for helping to settle the baby down, you're really good at keeping him happy" or "I could hear you singing in church this morning – you do have a beautiful voice" or "That back-rub you gave me felt great – you have really strong hands."

- **Be as specific as possible when you praise something about your child.** Saying "you're a good boy" doesn't mean very much. It also helps to express your feelings rather than make a blanket statement about some aspect of your child's accomplishments. You could say, for example, "I love the colors in that picture, they really make me think of an autumn day near the cottage" rather than, "That's a very good picture."

The more things you can give your child to feel positive about, the less important his weight will be in determining his overall level of self-esteem.

Help Your Child Meet Other Children and Adults Who Are Overweight and Feel Comfortable with Their Body Size

One researcher found that overweight children rarely choose each other as friends and in fact seem to actively avoid each other. It was speculated that the overweight children don't want to be classified as "the overweight gang" or "those fatties"; they feel that two or three large people together will attract more attention than one among a group of thinner children.

This is unfortunate, though, because children can benefit by knowing others who are facing similar problems. For adults, the social side of groups such as Weight Watchers is often very valuable. They meet others who are overweight and discover that they are interesting, charming, intelligent, accomplished people – demolishing all the myths that they might have worried about.

But children will rarely join groups designed to help them lose weight. One public health unit attempted to start a group for overweight school-age children, but none of the children who fit their classifications would attend. It was simply too embarrassing for them.

So how can you help your overweight child feel less alone with his concerns? Look in your own family first. You probably have relatives who are also larger than average.

For Jake, talking to his Uncle Mike was a big help. "I knew Jake was feeling really bad about his weight, so I asked Mike to talk to him," says Jake's father. "Mike's always been big, but he's always felt okay about it. The next time he came over, he took Jake for a walk – and when they came back, Jake had a big smile on his face."

Jake told his dad, "You know what Uncle Mike does every morning when he wakes up? He stands in front of the mirror with no clothes on and he says 'Perfect!' That's what I'm going to do, too!"

Of course, this didn't eliminate all the teasing in Jake's life, and he had many more walks with his Uncle Mike to talk about his concerns. But it started him along a road to more positive feelings about himself.

You could also invite some of your child's larger-size classmates or acquaintances from other activities to parties and other events at your house (with your child's permission, of course).

Even just seeing larger-size people who are receiving awards or accomplishing important things will help your child become aware of the diversity of sizes in our world. Television and movies can give the very misleading impression that everyone is thin – even in talk show audiences, the people are deliberately seated so that the thinner ones are in the front rows. But you can easily find photos of talented writers, musicians, artists and other successful larger-than-average people, and take the time to point them out to your family.

Helena went with her family to the National Arabian Horse Championships held in a town near her home. Although she loved horses, she had been hesitating about doing much riding because she felt too fat. She didn't look anything like the riders she'd seen in movies and on television.

To her surprise and delight, the National Championship in one class went to a horse ridden by a very large woman. Helena applauded vigorously and said to her mother, "Fat people can win in horse shows! Can I start taking riding lessons?" Her mother was thrilled to hear Helena's request and promised to enroll her in classes as soon as possible.

It's important for children to know that being overweight doesn't have to keep them from accomplishing things they want to do and from being happy, successful people.

Encourage His or Her Social Life by Inviting Friends Over

Many overweight children have no social problems, but some find they have few friends and difficulty in making new ones. Some are afraid even to try because they don't want to face teasing and rejection.

You can help by making your home a welcoming place for your child's friends and by encouraging her to invite other children over. When children are in your home, they are less likely to tease your child, and if they do, you can quickly intervene. You will also have a chance to observe how your child interacts with her friends and decide if she needs some help in learning social skills.

Suggest she begin by inviting a friend over after school. As the parent, your job is just to provide snacks and a comfortable place to play. If that goes well, you can encourage her to invite a group of friends over on another occasion – and there are all kinds of possible get-together occasions from birthdays to Hallowe'en or back-to-school parties. Help her to be creative in thinking of fun activities to do with friends and contribute as many of your own ideas as possible.

If you are going out for a family activity (anything from a visit to the library to swimming at the local pool) and you have room, encourage your child to invite a friend or two to join you. Is there a classmate on the route she takes to school who might be willing to walk with her, at least part way? Does your child have any special interests or hobbies – music, art, sports? Taking lessons or joining a team at school can help him or her to meet other children with similar interests – one of the best ways to make friends.

Too many adults put their social lives on hold until they lose weight – and too often that day never comes. Help your child to develop friendships and recognize that her weight is not a barrier to satisfying relationships.

You probably can't eliminate teasing from your overweight child's life but, after all, teasing is part of life for most children. What you can do is offer lots of loving support and encouragement to help your child feel strong enough to cope with it and keep his or her self-esteem intact.

5

Increasing Activity

When Anna's family made the move from the city to the country, she was ten and had been overweight most of her life. When she wasn't at school, she had spent her days watching TV or playing with friends on the same block. But she loved horses and other animals and was eager to move to the farm – she'd been promised a horse of her own and the family was planning to get a dog as well.

The change in environment meant some big changes in Anna's life. Now she got up early to feed her horse and the other animals before she went off to school, and she usually took her puppy for a morning walk as well. After school she hurried out to the barn to groom her horse and she rode every day when the weather permitted. Then after supper the puppy needed another walk, and on the weekend Anna cleaned out the stalls and rode to neighboring farms to visit her friends.

Six months after the move, Anna noticed that she was becoming slimmer. The funny thing was, she figured out that she was actually eating more than she had before – all that outdoor work before breakfast seemed to give her a hearty appetite when she finally got back in the house. She usually asked her mother to pack two sandwiches for lunch now, instead of one. All the same, she was definitely thinner and more muscular than she had been.

Two years later, when Anna started puberty, she went through another plump stage, but when she began to grow quickly she slimmed down again. She continued to work around the farm, ride almost every day and take her dog for frequent walks, and her weight remained in the average range.

Anna's story shows quite vividly how our activity level affects our weight. In fact, the research shows that activity is probably the most important area for those who want to reduce their weight, particularly children.

Let's look at the average day of an average North American boy, age nine.

7:00 a.m.	Wakes up. Washes face, brushes teeth, combs hair, gets dressed. Prepares a bowl of cereal and eats it in front of the TV.
7:50 a.m.	Walks to corner to catch school bus. Rides 25 minutes to school.
8:15 a.m.	Arrives 5 minutes before the bell rings, greets friends and talks until time to go into class.
8:25 to 10:15	Works at his desk in the classroom.
10:15 to 10:30	Morning recess. First has to tidy up desk, put on coat, line up with other students before going into playground. This uses up at least 5 minutes of recess time, more if the teacher decides the children aren't behaving and makes them stand in the line longer. Plays outside for about 10 minutes, climbing on equipment or playing ball. On rainy days, teacher holds indoor recess and children stay at their desks.
10:30 to 12:00	Works at his desk.
12:00 to 12:15	Eats lunch.

12:15 to 12:45   Outside in playground if weather is good. The more athletic kids often play sports, but many kids – especially those who are overweight – are excluded from this. Girls in particular may just stand around talking.

12:45 to 2:30   Works at his desk.

2:30 to 3:15   Today is one of three gym classes scheduled each week at this child's school. They're learning to do vaults over a gymnastics-style horse. That means they spend most of their time in line, waiting for their turns to run briefly across the gym and jump over the horse.

3:20 p.m.   School is dismissed. He walks to the school bus and is driven home.

3:45 p.m.   Older sister is babysitting and she already has the TV on. He settles down with a snack to watch until Mom and Dad get home from work.

5:30 p.m.   Mom's home. She starts preparing supper. The kids continue watching TV.

6:30 p.m.   The TV goes off while the family eats supper. The kids load the dishwasher, then gather up their homework to do in front of the TV.

8:30 p.m.   Time for a bath, and then a snack before bedtime.

9:00 p.m.   In bed with a book to read before he falls asleep.

That's a pretty typical day in an ordinary family and it's easy to see that there isn't a lot of exercise involved. How can we improve it? How can we include activity in our daily routines?

Perhaps the first question parents will ask is: How much activity is necessary? We don't know for sure. Some studies of normal weight people have suggested that the body begins burning fat after 20 minutes of aerobic exercise. (Aerobic exercise is continuous movement that raises the heart rate but still allows the person to speak comfortably.) But at least one study of overweight women found that these women needed to exercise for at least one hour daily as well as reduce the number of calories they ate in order to lose weight. We do know, though, that almost any increase in activity will help your child become fitter, stronger and more muscular.

You don't have to move to the country to help your child become more active. There are many small changes you can make in your daily routine that will make a significant difference when they are added up.

First of all, don't ever make exercising a negative experience. If eating is a reward and exercising a punishment, you are almost guaranteeing that your child will continue to be overweight. The gym teachers who say that the last child to complete a circuit of the track has to do 50 pushups are doing just the opposite of what they intend. They're teaching the child that exercise is something bad, something they should do everything they can to avoid.

Exercise and activity can and should be fun. That's why it's important to start slowly and gently. The overweight and inactive child is particularly vulnerable to injury. He might also feel uncoordinated and awkward if he isn't used to a lot of physical activity. Those muscles have to get used to working.

Telling your child "You need the exercise" before sending him on a walk or into some activity is insulting and sets up negative feelings about the activity. We all need exercise. It's good for thin people as well as heavier people. Make the goal to increase activity a family goal, not just something the overweight child is expected to do because of his "problem."

What kinds of exercise are most valuable for overweight children? First of all, remember that any exercise is good. Even a few minutes of walking is better than spending those few minutes watching TV, for example. But some kinds of exercise are more helpful than others.

Moderate exercise burns fat – exactly what you want it to do – while more intense exercise will burn sugars from the bloodstream (as well as increasing the risk of injury). How do you know you are exercising moderately? For adults, fitness instructors usually explain how to calculate a target heart rate based on the person's age. Moderate aerobic exercise raises the heart rate to a certain percentage of that range.

These calculations are a bit too complicated for most children. Instead, check to see if the child can still talk comfortably while doing the exercise. He should feel that his heart is beating faster, but not be puffing and unable to talk because of the exertion.

Exercise that uses **large body muscles** is also most likely to be good for burning fat. That means the muscles in your arms and legs, used in activities like swimming and walking. Situps can tighten stomach muscles but won't go very far in helping to reduce fat.

Another important fact to remember is that muscles use up more calories than fat even at rest. As increased activity builds more muscle while reducing fat, your child will develop a faster metabolism and a tendency to be thinner.

Sustained exercise is also important. Our imaginary child's 10 minutes of running around the playground will burn up a few calories and give him a chance to work off some of the stress of being in school, but it won't do much to keep his weight from going up. It takes time to use enough calories to affect weight.

It isn't likely that children will need to exercise as long as some overweight adults to have the desired results, but planning for sustained exercise is the best approach. Aim for at least 20 to 30 minutes and go for longer times if possible. This will lead to muscle conditioning as well as energy use.

Increasing activity is important. But how do you nudge your non-athletic, TV-addicted child in that direction without creating a lot of resentment and unhappiness?

It can be done.

The first step is to think of this as a change for the whole family. You can all benefit from adding more activity and exercise to your life (many thin people are actually in rather poor physical condition), so don't put the focus on your overweight child (or children). Join in!

Secondly, consider the three areas of your child's daily life and the changes that can be made to increase her activity level *painlessly*.

At Home

For the last hundred years or so, we have concentrated on making our daily lives more convenient and less physically demanding. Few people hang clothes out on a line any more – now we just transfer them from the washer to the dryer. Most people have dishwashers to clean up after meals instead of doing dishes by hand. If we need to go to the store or our kids need to go somewhere special, we hop in the car and get there in minutes.

The result is that while we may be able to get a great deal more done each day than our ancestors could accomplish, we are also getting, on average, much less physical exercise.

Here are more than fifty ways to make your child's everyday life more active. Some involve money, but others are free. Pick those that suit your family and let this list inspire you to think of your own creative and active ideas.

1. Buy him a dog that needs to be walked at least twice a day.
2. Ask her to mail all your letters – walking there and back.
3. Cancel your newspaper subscription and have him go out to buy you a paper each day.
4. Park at the far end of the parking lot when you go to the mall.
5. Walk to the store together if you can.
6. Don't take the elevator or the escalator when you can go up or down the stairs, even if it takes a bit longer.
7. Buy rollerblades for your child and let him skate around the basement or an empty parking lot.
8. Put up a basketball net in your driveway or backyard and get a basketball.
9. Hang a trapeze, swings, rings, rope, etc. from your basement ceiling. Use an old mattress underneath for safety.
10. Get a small rebounder trampoline and leave it near the TV set.
11. Make going to the park for a walk a family ritual.

12. When you buy groceries, have the kids bring them in from the car and put them away.

13. Make a kite together, then go fly it. You hold it up, while she runs ahead to make it catch the breeze.

14. If he thinks walking is "too hard," let him ride his bike alongside you while you walk.

15. Assign her the outdoor chores, which tend to be more active: sweeping the walk, shoveling the driveway, raking the yard.

16. Allow TV-watching time *if* he rides the exercise bike (set up in front of the TV) while watching.

17. On rainy days, dress appropriately and go for a walk in the rain.

18. On the days when you've planned to have dessert, walk somewhere to get it (an ice cream cone or cookie treat) and then walk home again.

19. Make ice cream the old-fashioned way, with lots of churning.

20. Bake bread together and let him do the kneading.

21. Grow a garden and let her do the digging, weeding and harvesting. (This also tends to encourage the eating of home-grown vegetables.)

22. If you like background music around the house, play lively songs so the kids feel like moving.

23. Have a family dancing party to celebrate something (or nothing at all).

24. Go to the library, parking as far away as possible, and borrow lots of heavy books.

25. Plan active summer vacations and day trips: hiking marked trails in conservation areas, swimming, horseback riding, biking.

26. Plan active winter vacations: a walking tour of the Christmas lights in your neighborhood, cross-country skiing, swimming in indoor pools.

27. Go to a Christmas tree farm where you can walk out into the woods, cut down your own tree and drag it back to the car.

28. Hide the remote control for the TV so he has to at least get up and change channels.

29. If you have a fireplace, put her in charge of bringing in the wood (she could also chop it if she's old enough).

30. Ask him to take his baby brother or sister or neighbor's baby for a daily walk (join him if possible).

31. Buy a swim pass to your community pool and use it frequently.

32. If you have to drive him to school, drop him off several blocks away.

33. Plan no-car weekends when the entire family walks or bikes everywhere (this is good for the environment, too).

34. Make family environmental rules about using the car: for example, only for trips of more than six blocks. For shorter trips, people have to walk or ride bikes.

35. Use a clothesline instead of the dryer and have your child help hang out the clothes and bring them in.

36. Play follow-the-leader, and include lots of skips, jumps and runs.

37. Have a family scavenger hunt that involves everyone running around the neighborhood looking for various items.

38. Give your child massages – they will relax muscles and stimulate the circulation.

39. Plan lively birthday parties – take the kids to play miniature golf, rent a pool for an hour or go to a local gymnastics club.

40. For at-home birthdays, include lots of active games such as tag, statues or musical chairs.

41. Enter fundraising walk-a-thons in your community. Even if you only have one or two sponsors (and even if it's just you every time), they'll be glad to have your child take part.

42. Buy strap-on ankle and wrist weights that the child can wear around the house during his normal activities.

43. Or let her carry a couple of tin cans while she exercises.

44. If he's interested in any of the exercise videos, consider buying one – but remember that most are simply not geared to children. Try one of the learn-to-dance videos that feature country music, if you think that might be more appealing.

45. When you're downstairs, ask her to get you the things you need from upstairs.

46. Help him get a paper route or a job delivering flyers in your neighborhood. This will combine regular exercise with a chance to earn extra money.

47. Rearrange your household furniture frequently – with your child's help (this is fun anyway).

48. Ask him to take out the garbage and the recycling box each week. Take other garbage out to your community dump and let him carry it to the right bin.

49. Choose active rewards for good behavior or special achievements. You might reward a successful school project with a visit to the batting cages or an hour of horseback riding or just a walk through a favorite park.

50. Encourage active play on children's playgrounds. School-age kids often feel too old for swings and slides, but many playgrounds now have a variety of activities that suit all ages. If they feel embarrassed, ask them to take a younger sibling or neighborhood child on the equipment.

51. Go for barefoot walks in the sand.

52. Go for walks at night. Just being able to stay up late is a treat for most kids, and walks in the dark are special – you can look for stars and for animals that appear only at night.

53. Get a skipping rope and teach her all the skipping games you knew as a child.

At School

All schools, of course, have some kind of gym program during which children can be active. Unfortunately, you can't rely on these classes to meet your child's need for exercise.

Kanchana's fifth grade class is scheduled to have gym class three times a week. They can't use it any more often because the school only has one gymnasium and the other classes also need their scheduled gym time. The focus of the school physical education curriculum is on learning skills used in various sports, so most gym classes are divided between teacher instruction on a specific technique and time for the students to practice what they have learned. Kanchana changes into gym clothes at the beginning of each class, but she's rarely sweaty when the class ends.

Some of those three classes each week are used up by health classes, when the students learn about good nutrition, the hazards of smoking and other important topics. For those sessions, the class usually sits on the gym floor while the teacher talks or shows a movie. Other classes are pre-empted by assemblies or special programs.

Sometimes during gym class the teacher organizes games: volleyball, basketball, dodge ball. Kanchana hates those most of all. The teacher invariably picks two team captains and lets them choose sides; overweight children like Kanchana are always among the last to be picked. Then her captain tries to place her in the least important spot – which usually means the least active spot as well. Since she already feels humiliated about being picked last, she isn't inclined to put a lot of effort into the game. Most of the time she just stands around wondering if the ball will ever come her way.

The school has several sports teams that practice during lunch and sometimes after school, but Kanchana wouldn't even consider going out for one of those. She's afraid the other kids would laugh at her for even trying, and she's pretty sure she wouldn't be good enough to make the team. She spends her lunch hours talking with the other girls on the playground.

David's teacher – who has had a weight problem most of his life and knows what a struggle it can be – has taken a different approach.

His class is also scheduled into the gym three times a week, but he doesn't think that's enough. Every morning, before beginning the classroom work, he takes all his students for a half-hour march around the schoolyard and neighborhood. He finds it keeps them calmer during the day, too, when they've had this chance to work off their energy.

Your child is probably spending six or more hours every day in school, and much of that time is sitting down at a desk. How can you work with your school to increase the amount of exercise the children get?

Here are some suggestions you might make to your child's teacher or the school's principal:

1. A lunchtime exercise class can be fun for staff and students. Perhaps a teacher or interested parent might be willing to organize it and include aerobic dancing or walks around the community.

2. School teams can be organized that involve and include all children, no matter how athletic they are. At Jay's school, for example, all children were automatically assigned to a house team, and games in various sports were arranged every day during the lunch hour. The teams got points for every member who showed up, as well as for winning the game – and sometimes the "losing" team actually got more points than the winners! At the end of the year, awards were given out for participation as well as accomplishments.

3. Talk to the teacher about the curriculum for the physical education program. If the gym is not always available, perhaps it could be supplemented with walks in the schoolyard or to other community locations.

4. Suggest activity-oriented field trips. It's great to go to museums and art galleries, but many teachers also incorporate outings to a skating rink, swimming pool, gymnastics club or other local facility into their yearly plan. If you know about one that your child might like, drop the teacher a note.

5. You can make similar suggestions to the school board. Where Teresa lives, for example, every third grade child gets weekly swimming lessons at no cost to the parents. This is good exercise and also teaches the child some very important water-safety skills.

6. Attend PTA meetings and encourage the organization to make fitness for all students a priority. It's important not to single out the heavier children for these activities – exercise is valuable for everyone.

7. Find out what your child's teacher likes to do – if she's a runner, the kids could run three or four mornings a week. Her other activities may also be incorporated into class activities (as long as it isn't hang gliding!).

When staff are interested, the school can be a terrific way of introducing children to new activities and incorporating exercise into their daily routines. If you are finding it difficult to work with your school, concentrate on increasing activity levels at home or through other activities.

Lenore Kilmartin is homeschooling her four children and has discovered many ways to help them keep fit even though they have no gymnasium and their day is quite unstructured.

"One of my goals each day," she says, "is to go for a walk with all the children. It might be in the morning or it might be in the afternoon, but I try to fit it in somewhere."

Lenore has also banded together with other homeschooling parents to find recreational activities for their children. They have arranged with a community church to use a large playroom on Friday mornings, and they arrive with balls and other equipment for the children to use in games and sports. A local gymnastics club sat largely unused during the school day and was pleased to offer inexpensive lessons for the homeschooling kids; a nearby swimming pool made similar arrangements with Lenore and her friends.

"It's really worked out very well," Lenore says. "I consider the physical side of my children's education as important as the academic side, and homeschooling really makes it easy to do both."

Lenore finds that even without formal instruction, the children are eager to use the equipment or to swim in the pool and get plenty of exercise through their play activities.

Organized Sports and Activities

Leah saw her first ballet at age four and she fell in love with dancing. Although her rounded figure wasn't the typical ballerina's physique, her parents enrolled her in ballet classes when she was five and she loved them. She stayed plump despite the dancing, but never minded – until she turned ten.

The ballet school was auditioning for their annual performance and after five years of training Leah felt ready. She knew the steps and the techniques. But she wasn't given even a small part – because, the teacher explained, she wouldn't fit into any of the costumes.

Leah knew what her teacher meant. She was too fat. She'd heard the other girls – already much thinner than her – complaining about being too heavy and discussing their diets. Her passion for ballet began to fade and a year later she quit taking lessons altogether.

Iain signed up for baseball because his parents were urging him to take up a sport of some kind and baseball was his favorite. He loved to watch the game on TV. The league he joined was a good one; each child was guaranteed to play a certain amount of time and no one was left sitting on the bench.

Unfortunately, baseball is simply not a very active game. There will be brief moments of running after a hit ball or racing around the bases, followed by long periods of standing in the outfield wondering if the ball will ever come this way or sitting in the lineup waiting for your turn at bat. Iain was never a spectacular player, but he enjoyed baseball and signed up again the next season. He had fun, but it did nothing to improve his fitness levels or reduce his weight.

Organized sports, dancing and other activities can, at first, seem like a terrific way to increase a child's exercise level and reduce his or her weight. And they can be both fun and beneficial. However, there are a few pitfalls to be aware of:

Some Sports Are Not Very Good Exercise

To succeed in a sport like baseball, you need to be physically fit, but you won't likely get that way playing the game. Most professional players include a vigorous exercise routine as part of their training besides actually playing the game. (Of course, some don't – remember Babe Ruth?) Golf is another example of a not-very-active sport, especially when you ride in a golf cart between the holes.

Remember our definitions of the best kind of activities for overweight children from the beginning of this chapter? The emphasis should be on sustained, moderate movement. Any sport that has only brief bursts of running, jumping or other exercise will simply not be sufficient to increase the child's fitness level and promote weight loss.

Be sure to watch an actual game of the sport you are considering, if you are not already familiar with it, before signing up your child. Are most of the children moving throughout most of the game? Are they sweaty and maybe breathing a bit hard afterwards (although preferably not exhausted)?

Some good choices: horseback riding, soccer, hockey, ice-skating, basketball, cross-country skiing, swimming, running and any others that involve continuous movement.

Some Teams Encourage Only the Best Players to Play

It won't do your child any good at all to be part of a team in an active sport like soccer if she spends most of the season sitting on the bench. The overweight child may not even get much chance to demonstrate what he can do, because the coach may assume he's no good because of his size. And of course, many overweight children do find that they are physically a bit awkward or uncoordinated and therefore even more likely to be left on the sidelines.

Before you sign up, ask both the league or organization and the coach about the policy on playing time. Some leagues insist on a strict rotation schedule, so that every child gets to play the same amount of time. This is ideal. Others leave playing time up to the discretion of the individual coach, so there may be considerable variation between one team and another.

Remember that it is far more important for your child to be actively involved and playing the game than to be part of a winning team but sitting on the bench most of the time.

Highly Competitive Teams or Activities Can Be Very Damaging to Your Child's Self-Esteem

Like the little girl who dropped out of ballet because she was never given any parts in the school's productions, it can be very hurtful to a child to work hard during class but then be excluded from the shows because of his or her size.

At Teresa's daughter's ballet school, the staff are committed to including all their students in performances. They have been quite creative in adding parts with costumes that disguise the overweight child's size and yet make an interesting and entertaining addition to the show. For example, heavier dancers have had parts as battling mice, maids and housekeepers, and Russian dancers in the school's annual performance of *The Nutcracker*.

When teams are focused on winning, it can sometimes be at the expense of the less-athletic child. One boy tells about playing on a soccer team with a league that insisted all children play the same amount of time during each game. But when his team reached the finals, the coach called him at home and asked him not to come to the next game. Then the coach would be able to play his more talented players for a longer time and increase the team's chances of winning the championship. The coach saw this as an appeal to the boy's sense of team spirit – encouraging him to make a small sacrifice to help the rest of the team win. But for the boy, it was devastating. He saw himself as a hindrance to the team, not a help, and he never played soccer again.

Parents should also be aware that some teachers or coaches place a high value on thinness, especially in dance, gymnastics and figure skating. A child who is only slightly plump may be the target of constant comments about her weight, encouragement to diet and sometimes even threats – "If you don't lose some weight, you won't be able to compete next month." This can be damaging to the child's health as well as her self-esteem.

You Must Match the Sport with the Child

The reasons why we like one sport or activity and not another are often mysterious. Why is Brian absolutely passionate about soccer and Joyce a dedicated baseball fan? What inspired Lisa at age four to devote herself to ballet? It's hard to say. Most of us are physically better suited for some activities than for others, but it may take some experimenting to find out which is right for us.

Teresa's friend Susan, noticing Lisa's dedication to dancing, once asked Teresa, "How did you make Lisa be so interested in ballet? I'd like to get my daughter to be like that." Well, "making a child be interested" is a hopeless goal. Ballet takes a lot of discipline and hard work, and no child is likely to stick with it unless he or she has made an internal choice to do so.

Overweight children, in particular, may resist being part of an organized sport. They see themselves as unathletic and (quite reasonably) worry about being teased or left out.

How can you help them get involved? Some tips:

- Watch for and encourage any spark of interest. Does your child have good eye-hand co-ordination? Perhaps he'd like to try tennis or another racket sport. Does your daughter like horses? Maybe horseback riding would be a good choice. Be alert for opportunities to suggest new sports.

- Individual sports may be better than team sports, and lessons may be better than competitive activities. Joseph is quite overweight and will never be a gymnastics star, but he thoroughly enjoys his weekly lesson at the community gymnastics club and at home he often practices the tumbling and other skills he has learned. He's noticed that he's getting stronger and developing more muscles. The club coaches are extremely supportive of Joseph and praise his accomplishments without any concerns that he's not as good as some of the other club members. However, their attitude might be very different if he were part of a competing team.

- Consider becoming involved yourself as a coach, assistant coach, scorekeeper or convener. Many leagues and schools rely on parent volunteers to keep running and your help will definitely be appreciated. It also gives you the opportunity to have some input into how the team is managed, to make sure that all children get a chance to play and to help create a positive and encouraging atmosphere.

- Less-common or unusual sports may also be good choices because there's likely to be less competition to participate. Your child may be intrigued by the idea of trying something that nobody else he knows is doing, whether it's tai chi, fencing, race-walking, dressage or rock-climbing.

- Karate, judo and other martial arts or even wrestling may seem more appealing to boys or girls who see themselves as not particularly athletic. The idea of becoming strong and able to defend themselves can encourage them to work hard at these activities.

- Let your child quit if it's not working out. Sometimes, especially after having paid a hefty fee to enroll a child in sports or other lessons, parents are reluctant to let the child drop out if he discovers he hates it. The unfortunate side-effect of insisting that the child continue can be that he then refuses to try anything new because he's afraid of being stuck in the activity even if he doesn't like it.

Accept that your child (this applies to all children, but even more so to an overweight child) may need to try many different activities before finding one that is right for him or her. Try to arrange to pay for a short trial period, if possible, and look on the course or team as an experiment, not a commitment.

If your child decides to drop out, try to find out exactly why she's unhappy with the activity. Is it the teacher or coach, the philosophy of the school, one other kid in the class or just that the activity isn't right for her? The answers to those questions will help you make better decisions next time. Always let her know that she can try soccer, or ballet, or bowling again in a few months or a few years if she wants.

For some children, organized sports and lessons are a great way to increase their activity level. Finding the right team or class, though, can be a challenge for the overweight child.

FAMILY SPORTS

Organized sports often appeal to parents because they seem easy. Pay your fee, drop the child off at the practice and pick him up later. They don't have to take part or help their child learn the skills. For many busy families, it seems impossible to do more.

And yet there are real advantages to adding family sports to your schedule. You eliminate the problems of insensitive or discouraging coaches who can make life difficult for your child and you increase the fitness of everyone in your family as well as the overweight child or children.

The activities you choose, of course, will depend on your family size, where you live, how much money you have to spend and what your interests are. The Kennedys had enough children and enough space to make touch-football games a family tradition, but most of us have more limitations on our sports. Here are some easy suggestions:

Hiking is one of the easiest activities to get started in. All you need are sturdy hiking boots for every member of the family (and you can probably get away with running shoes for short walks) and comfortable clothes. (Good shoes that provide lots of support and clothes that don't chafe or bind and are comfortably loose are essential for the overweight child.)

The Pitman family lives near the Crawford Lake Conservation area, which features a restored Native village and a lake surrounded by a boardwalk. When the children were small, we walked around the lake twice each time we visited. Now that they are older, we've begun exploring the trails and paths that lead through the conservation area. These are easy hikes, the trails are well marked and we know exactly how long each path is. The views are spectacular and it's a lot of fun.

Other families get involved in wilderness hiking in a more ambitious way. There are many hiking clubs eagerly looking for new members or trails that can be explored inexpensively.

You don't even have to leave the city to go for a hike. In some cities, for example, a number of major parks are linked together and provide a terrific hiking route. You can also "hike" right through your town, exploring major streets and side streets. The scenery won't be the same, and you probably won't have many hills to climb, but these kinds of expeditions can still be fun as well as good exercise.

The important thing is to start slowly. If your overweight child comes home from his first hike with blisters and sore, aching muscles, he isn't likely to go out on a second hike. At Crawford Lake, for example, the trails are marked according to the level of difficulty and we started with the easiest one. Don't be afraid to turn back if the trail is getting too steep or your child is feeling too tired. You can probably go farther next time.

And make the hikes enjoyable. Some children appreciate the quiet beauties of nature more than others, so look for hikes that will appeal to everyone. Our favorite Crawford Lake trail ends with a view from high up on the Niagara Escarpment where you can look across the countryside for miles and miles. However, you might find a hike through town works better for a child who finds nature boring, especially if you can do some window shopping or pass by a construction site on the way.

Finally, don't forget to schedule your family hikes as regular, planned events. Going for a walk once in a while won't help you very far along toward your goal of increased fitness.

Biking can be a great alternative if just walking along seems too slow for your family. The increasing popularity of biking is demonstrated by the bike paths that have been created in many cities and towns. Your local library probably carries several books describing bike trips in the area around your community.

Overweight children often find biking is easier and more enjoyable for them than walking. When they walk or run, their thighs often rub together, causing blisters or an uncomfortable rash. Their weight also may mean their feet and legs hurt more when they walk. Both of these problems vanish when using a bike. You will need to make sure you pick a bike that fits your child comfortably, particularly the seat. Many bike seats are designed for small, athletic bums and will only cause your heavier child to feel miserable and hate biking. Take some time to try out several bikes in order to get just the right one.

If you decide to take up biking as a family, pay attention to the safety issues. Helmets are essential for everyone (yes, parents need to wear them, too). Small children should be carried in approved safety seats or towed behind the bike in a bike buggy (these are actually safer than the seats because they keep the child close to the ground) and they should wear helmets, too. Go over the rules of the road with your older children and be sure they know how to ride safely before starting out on any longer trips.

Just as with hiking, it's important to start slowly. One family decided to travel to Massachusetts and go on a biking holiday with their two children. They flew out and rented bikes on their arrival, but they only lasted two days before they gave in and rented a car instead. While the parents were fairly fit, they'd forgotten that biking uses different muscles, and all four of them were really suffering from the new activity.

So begin with short trips around your neighborhood. A nightly bike ride can be good preparation for a longer weekend trip, and a few months of regular cycling is a good way to prepare for a week-long biking holiday.

Horseback riding, while expensive, is a great family activity. Horses (like people) come in all shapes and sizes, so you can probably find one to suit every family member. And it is one sport in which the heavier child may feel he or she can participate equally.

We described in an earlier chapter the experience of Helena, who was delighted to see an overweight rider win a championship ribbon at a horse show she attended. Though many riders are slender, the shows are judged on each horse's performance, and many heavier riders bring home their share of ribbons. That can be a real boost to an overweight child who feels he simply can't compete in most sports.

While it may seem that the child is being carried by the horse, riding is, in fact, good exercise. The rider is rarely passive – it takes a lot of work just to stay in the saddle and control the horse, and as the rider's skill level increases, so does the amount of exercise. (If you doubt this, just notice how your arm and leg muscles feel the day after a ride.)

Working with a live animal can also be good for your child's self-esteem. Horses respond to affection and gentle treatment and don't judge people by appearances. Many children discover a real bond with horses and enjoy helping out with the barn chores (yes, more exercise) as well as the actual riding.

Cross-country skiing can be a great activity that helps your family get through the winter. It's excellent exercise, can be done at any speed and doesn't have the risk or expense of downhill skiing.

Some parts of the country don't have enough snow in winter to make this practical. Other communities lack open parks or trails where people can ski, although there are usually regional or provincial parks with ski trails at minimal cost.

The problem for the overweight child may be in finding a good ski suit that fits. Most are designed for thinner children and you might be better off buying a separate jacket and snow pants to get the best fit. Proper clothing is essential. Cross-country skiing also requires some co-ordination and the heavier child may feel awkward at first. A few lessons might be helpful; the skills aren't difficult to learn and the rewards of gliding across the snowy country quickly make the initial effort worthwhile.

Remember to pace yourself according to your child's abilities. Plan a route that doesn't take you too far away from home base at first, so you can return if your child gets tired. Cross-country skiing uses muscles that don't get much exercise in most daily activities, so your child may be stiff and sore pretty quickly. You might try buying an indoor ski exerciser that could be used to strengthen those ski muscles between outings.

Swimming is an excellent exercise that is particularly good for those who are overweight or out of shape, because there is little risk of injury as there might be in running or aerobic dancing. When you are swimming, the water supports your weight, so you aren't putting a lot of stress on bones or muscles.

Most adults who are swimming to increase fitness will do laps; the continuous, moderate exertion that helps burn fat is probably best achieved that way. However, most children think laps are boring and the overweight child may prefer to just float in the water and relax. Not much exercise in that!

Swimming lessons are rarely helpful in increasing the child's actual activity level. They usually focus on teaching specific skills (diving, kicking) and often the children spend a fair amount of time sitting on the side waiting while the instructor demonstrates something or watches another child perform.

That's why swimming is most beneficial when it's undertaken as a family activity. Playing games in the water can keep your child active and he'll barely notice he's exercising. Try pool volleyball or basketball, tag or fetching items from the bottom of the pool. Maybe the children would like to make up their own synchronized swimming routines to music.

Swimming is sometimes more expensive than activities like walking that just require a good pair of shoes. But many communities offer swim passes or less-expensive books of tickets at the public pools. You might be able to join your local Y; if money is a problem, most Y's will reduce or even eliminate membership fees.

Your biggest obstacle may be the discomfort your child feels about being seen in a bathing suit. We ourselves sometimes long for the days when bathing suits covered the body from neck to knees – maybe they were harder to swim in, but at least nobody felt embarrassed about being seen in one! Some suggestions:

- Help your child find the most flattering bathing suit possible. Many girls' suits come with little skirts and front panels designed to make the child feel less self-conscious. A heavy boy might prefer a suit in a loose, boxer short or "jammer" style rather than a brief style.

- Ask if your child can swim with a T-shirt on as well as his or her bathing suit. At some pools, this is forbidden (though we have no idea why) but others don't mind. Many overweight children who would never be seen in public in a bathing suit feel comfortable swimming with a T-shirt on too.

- Take your child along to the pool just to watch. She'll see swimmers of all shapes and sizes having a good time, and just knowing that she won't be the only heavier person there might help her feel more relaxed about taking part.

Just Do It!

In our efforts to make life more convenient, we've somehow managed to make it both more stressful and less active. We now have to consciously work to make sure we reach the activity level that was automatic a generation or two ago.

Let your child know that exercise is important in everyone's life and should be part of his or her plans every day. Look for ways to incorporate activity in everything you do. It's also essential to make these activities as much fun as possible, either by turning them into games or doing them as a group so that they become social activities. Once you see the rewards – a family where everyone is fitter, more energetic and happier – you'll be glad you made the effort.

Increasing activity is one key to becoming fitter. Healthy eating is the other part of the equation, and the next chapter will look at ways to help your child improve his or her eating habits.

6

Healthy Eating

While the research on body size and weight control is ongoing and the subject is quite complex, there are a few essential guidelines for the parents of an overweight child.

- Don't put your child on a diet. Diets that restrict calories or food intake will depress the child's metabolism and may cause nutrient deficiencies and make it likely that the child's problems will become even worse.

- Unless your child is very obese, you can help him maintain his weight until he "grows into it." This will be a slow process, so don't look for rapid changes.

- To achieve a desirable weight, your child's daily food intake should be low in fat and high in fiber. Fat should not be restricted in children under two years of age, and should be between 20 to 30 percent of total calories in older children.

- Eating lower-fat foods needs to be combined with a program to increase your child's daily activity level to build muscle and increase fitness.

Food Preferences

It's a busy Thursday evening and Teresa and her daughter Lisa are in the grocery store, fighting their way through the crowds of shoppers and carts. Lisa notices a display of food and turns to her mother, her eyes pleading "Can we have Brussels sprouts, please? We haven't had Brussels sprouts in ages! Please?"

Another woman stares at them in amazement. "I don't think I've ever heard a child beg for Brussels sprouts in my whole life."

That's Lisa. She comes home and asks for a salad for her after-school snack and fruit is her favorite dessert, not because she's been told it's good for her but simply because she likes it best. High-fat foods, such as meat, tend to make her feel ill and she doesn't eat them. Yes, she's quite slender and will probably always be that way.

Then there's her brother Jeremy. He likes salads, too, but his favorite is Caesar salad with generous amounts of dressing. He never begs for Brussels sprouts in the store – he's the one asking for chocolate bars, potato chips and popsicles. When he comes home from school hungry, he doesn't want a salad – he wants brownies. Yes, he's on the chubby side, and his tastebuds are encouraging it.

Where do our tastes come from? It's hard to say. Much of it seems to be inborn – the study of twins who were adopted at birth and raised separately discovered that, as adults, the twins had very similar tastes. They liked the same foods and had similar dislikes – if one hated peas, so did the other. Often these tastes were as distinct as a preference for the same brand of a particular food. Some children are definitely born with a sweet tooth and others never really develop a passion for sweet things.

Are children who love high-fat, high-calorie foods doomed to an endless struggle with their appetite and weight? Not necessarily. Tastes can be changed, although it's not always easy. When Teresa was a child, her family always drank whole milk and she loved it. When she grew up and married, she tasted skim milk for the first time and frankly thought it tasted disgusting – like water with a little white paint mixed in. She tried 2 percent milk and that too struck her as watery and unpalatable. So she tried a gradual approach. For a while, she mixed whole milk and 2 percent and, while not as rich and creamy as she might have liked, Teresa found it drinkable. Eventually she was able to drink regular 2 percent, then 1 percent and finally skim milk.

But it isn't just that Teresa has convinced herself that skim milk is better. She actually prefers it now; on those occasions when she is served 2 percent milk it seems unpleasantly thick and fatty. She can't even imagine drinking whole milk any more.

Other changes Teresa has made in her own eating habits have affected her the same way. For example, when she was younger, she ate traditionally large portions of meat – slabs of roast beef, thick burgers, a couple of pork chops. Now her family eats several meat-less meals each week and has only small portions when they do serve meat. She finds that, as a result, large amounts of meat (a typical restaurant serving, for example) seem unappetizing and sit heavily in her stomach. Miriam and her family are vegetarians.

It may not be so easy to change other tastes. Teresa still loves chocolate and even after she went for six months without eating any, still craved it (and loved it when she finally ate a piece). For-tunately, it isn't necessary to change everything about the way your overweight child eats. We hope these suggestions will help you improve your family's nutrition painlessly.

Talking It Over

Is your child concerned about his or her weight? Does he want to make some changes in his eating patterns? If so, it might be worth-while to sit down together and discuss this issue.

Many children, frustrated with their body image, immediately want to go on a crash diet. They will tell their parents that they want no breakfast, a handful of carrot sticks for lunch and just a salad for dinner. Not only is this diet impossible to maintain, it is danger-ously unhealthy, especially for growing children who have higher nutrient needs than adults.

Low-calorie diets will cause some weight loss. But the weight lost is water and muscle as well as fat, and the body reacts to this starvation experience by lowering its metabolism. In other words, it now burns calories at a lower rate than before. It also increases appetite in a desperate attempt to get more food into the system – often leading to binge eating. Your dieting child will soon find herself thinking about food constantly. Almost inevitably, the dieting person regains the weight lost and more besides. This time, though, the body percentage of fat is higher than it was before, because the lost muscle tissue is not replaced. And it is the percentage of body fat, not the actual weight, that has the most effect on health. Many adult dieters know this painful cycle of weight loss and gain. Children can be trapped by it, too.

So how do you change your child's diet in a healthy way? Your discussion should emphasize food as a positive thing – the essential source of nutrients and fuel for your child's body. Taking a slow route to achieving the desired weight will be much more successful and less risky than trying a quick-weight-loss approach.

Begin with the United States Department of Agriculture (USDA) Food Guide Pyramid (which can be obtained from your local health department). Tape a copy to your fridge door and go over it with your child. Some children will want to make a chart to check off the number of fruits and vegetables they've eaten each day, or to sit down with you once a week and use the guide to plan their menus. But if your child isn't interested in being that involved in the planning, don't force the issue.

Your goal should be to increase the amount of fiber in his or her diet and to decrease the fat so that between 20 and 30 percent of total calories in your child's diet comes from fat. Assessing this will probably require some label-reading, at least in the early stages. Remember that one gram of fat has nine calories, so if the label only gives the grams of fat, you can simply multiply it out. A child who is consuming about 1200 calories a day should have between 27 and 40 grams of fat. You should emphasize not what you are giving up but what you intend to increase: fruits, vegetables, whole grains.

What if your child, despite being overweight, isn't interested in discussing nutrition, the food guide pyramid or anything else?

Don't drop the whole idea. These changes in eating will benefit the entire family, so they are well worth making. Call a family meeting and talk about what you intend to do, without any mention of the overweight child or children. We'd recommend this way of handling your planned changes anyway, even if you and your child have met privately at an earlier time. Discuss the new research showing that eating more fruits and vegetables and less fat can protect people from many diseases including cancer and heart attacks. Nutrition is often taught in schools today, so you may get more support than you expect.

Following the food guide will not cause rapid or dramatic weight loss. But that shouldn't be your goal. Remember that with a growing child you don't want her actually to lose weight – you simply want her to maintain her weight until she grows into it. Remember, too, that the more slowly this relative weight loss happens, the more likely she will be able to maintain it.

The Bonnici family gathered together on New Year's Eve and set some fitness-related goals for the coming year. They created both family and individual goals and posted them on the fridge where everyone could see them.

Some of the family goals were:

- To have at least two meatless days each week.

- To go cross-country skiing once a week during the winter (they'd all received skis as Christmas presents).

- To serve a salad every day before dinner.

- To have fruit desserts during the week and other desserts only on weekends.

Some of the children's individual goals were:

- To drink more juice and water and less pop.

- To get up 20 minutes earlier in the morning to have time for a good breakfast and to avoid snacking on chips or chocolate bars in the middle of the morning.

- To stop eating in front of the TV set.

Of course, like all New Year's resolutions, not all of these goals were kept. But it was a good beginning, and the family reviews these decisions and how they're all doing on a regular basis.

Other good times for setting goals or making resolutions are at the beginning of the summer, the beginning of the school year or on birthdays. Take advantage of these natural times for planning ahead to make the changes in your family's diet that you see are necessary.

At the Grocery Store

There's good news in your supermarket. Healthy eating has become a trend, and "light" versions of many foods are now available that simply didn't exist even a few years ago. Take advantage of these to make your shopping and meal-planning easier.

When you go grocery shopping, look for foods that are low in fat, low in sugar and high in fiber. This combination will help your child adjust his or her weight gradually, give plenty of essential nutrients and still allow your child to feel full.

Let's take a guided tour around a typical supermarket and point out some products that might be good choices. Even though it can be more challenging to shop with a child – grocery stores are carefully arranged to encourage impulse buying – we would encourage you to bring your overweight child if possible. Let him give you input into what foods he would like, what new things he's willing to try and what he's not ready to give up yet. Plan this first shopping trip for a day when the stores are not too busy and you have plenty of time to read labels, discuss the relative merits of various foods and make choices you'll both be happy with.

THE MEAT DEPARTMENT

Meat in general is one of the higher-fat foods and most nutritionists feel that reducing the amount of meat in our diets would be beneficial in a number of ways. As you choose meat for your family, consider these ideas:

- Plan at least one meatless day each week and try gradually to increase this. Many families are becoming entirely or primarily vegetarian.

- Plan to serve smaller portions of meat. A piece of meat about the size of a deck of cards for each person is plenty. Choosing ground meat or boneless meat that you will slice yourself makes it easier for you to control the size of each serving than if you serve pork chops, chicken parts or pre-made burgers. When making casseroles that normally use two pounds of meat, try using one and a half pounds instead.

- Choose lower-fat meats. Ground turkey or chicken is usually lower in fat than ground beef or pork, and your family often can't tell the difference. Read the labels – many stores highlight low-fat meats. When buying beef, look for extra-lean ground beef or cuts with the fat well trimmed. Often the leaner cuts are less expensive but require longer, slower cooking.

- Choose more fish. Fish is not only lower in fat but has some important nutrients that help to reduce cholesterol levels. Avoid battered fish sticks, however, and buy plain frozen fillets or fresh fish instead.

- Be cautious when buying processed and sliced meats. Look for those labeled low-fat or read the label to see exactly what the fat content is. Many producers are now offering prepared sliced turkey, combined ham and turkey and low-fat ham slices. The more traditional bolognas and other meats tend to be very high in fat and are not a good choice.

- Avoid bacon, hot dogs and other high-fat meats, or serve them in small quantities – using bacon as a "seasoning" alongside an otherwise low-fat meal. If your child just loves hot dogs, look for lower-fat versions or try some of the vegetarian hot dogs now on the market. Some of these are quite tasty – and who could tell anyway, with all that ketchup, mustard and relish loaded on top?

The Dairy Section

Ah, dairy products! Think of all that sour cream, ice cream, whole milk, cream cheese, whipped cream…. The list goes on and on, and you just know all of them are high in fat. They must be, because they taste so good.

The good news is that dairy producers have made significant efforts in recent years to offer consumers low-fat products. This is probably one of the easiest areas in which to reduce fat, and the new products are so good that you're not likely to have any complaints.

Like many of us, you probably pick up the same items every week as you hurry through the grocery store. The dairy section is one area where it's really worth taking the time to scout out new products, read some labels and try some new things.

- Switch to a lower-fat milk. If you're drinking whole or 2 percent now, you may want to do this gradually. Try mixing the higher-fat milk with a lower-fat one at first and slowly decrease the amount of fat. Even as you continue drinking a higher-fat milk, you can easily switch to skim milk on breakfast cereal and in cooking. Eventually you will be able to enjoy skim milk (we promise), or at least one-half percent. Some dairies offer skim milk (and skimmed chocolate milk) made with a special non-fat thickener that is said to give it a richer, more creamy taste. Some kids love it, some don't – but it's worth a try.

- Buy low-fat or skim-milk cheese. You might need to experiment a little bit to find a brand you like, as some definitely have a better flavor than others. Some also don't melt well and therefore are not suitable for use in cooking or things like grilled cheese sandwiches.

- Choose strongly flavored cheeses (e.g., sharp cheddar) so that you need less to get the taste you want.

- Look for "light" cream cheese. This is still a fairly high-fat food, but if you eat a lot of cream cheese, switching will help.

- Instead of sour cream, buy skim-milk or low-fat yogurt. The taste is a little different, but it's still good and works well in recipes.

- Instead of whipping cream, buy the little packages of powder that can be mixed with skim milk and whipped up with your mixer to make a lower-fat dessert topping. Not quite as rich and tasty but it does add that touch of glamour to a plain bowl of peach slices.

- Look for calorie-reduced or low-fat margarines. You might have to try more than one brand before you discover one that your family likes. Plan to use a lot less of these spreads. If you're really hooked on the taste of butter, try a whipped butter that spreads more easily on bread and gives you that butter taste with fewer calories (because you use less). Also look for butter-flavored powders or similar products that can be mixed with water to add that buttery flavor to cooked vegetables.

- Yogurt and cottage cheese both come in low-fat or skim-milk versions that taste as good as the higher-fat versions. Both are even better mixed with fruit – but buy them plain and add your own fruit at home, as the premixed varieties usually have lots of added sugar.

- Ice cream can be replaced by ice milk, sherbets, water ices, gelati, popsicles and other frozen desserts. Consider getting an ice cream maker and creating your own treats with low-fat recipes. This is an important area to let your child make some choices – if you decide that ice cream is too high in fat and sugar, show him the wide selection of frozen desserts on display in any grocery freezer and let him choose. Popsicles, while high in sugar, have no fat; some companies are making juice popsicles that are nutritious as well as a treat. There are many specially labeled diet desserts as well that might appeal to your child.

Some families really treasure the taste of the richer ice creams and decide to limit them to small quantities on special occasions rather than eliminate them altogether. (Since these ice creams are generally quite expensive, it's easy to make that decision.) But make sure these limits affect the whole family, not just the overweight child who sits with a diet popsicle while everyone else enjoys Haagen-Dazs Double Chocolate Chunks.

GRAINS AND BREADS

High fiber should be your goal and standard here, and most white breads just don't make the grade. Fiber is important in weight control for two reasons: it helps you feel full so that you eat less, and it speeds up the passage of foods through the intestines so fewer calories are absorbed. It's also important in preventing many serious diseases and avoiding minor discomforts such as constipation.

Most whole grains are naturally high in fiber. Unfortunately, the traditional western diet relies on food processing to remove most of that fiber. So we have white flour, white bread, white rice – all almost fiber-free.

For healthier eating, go back to those whole grains. If you have always used white flour for baking, try mixing it with whole wheat flour and following the same recipes. When the whole wheat flour is 50 percent or less than the total, you will hardly even notice it. Try bread made with 60 percent whole wheat flour, available in many stores. Buy brown rice instead of white – it takes a bit longer to cook, but has a delicious flavor and better texture. Some other tips:

- Look for diet breads and high-fiber breads – most grocery stores carry several brands. Watch out for egg breads or challah, which tend to be higher in fat. Try rye breads, oatmeal breads and bran breads, all usually high in fiber.

- If you have time, consider making your own bread with whole wheat flour and minimal fat. It's easier than you might think, especially with a breadmaker or a food processor or mixer to do the kneading (or better yet, ask your child to knead the bread dough – it's great exercise and he'll love being involved).

- Be very choosy about breakfast cereals. Some are incredibly high in fat and sugar. We love the TV commercials that suggest these cereals can be "part of a balanced breakfast" – note that the breakfast shown usually includes juice, fruit, toast and a muffin and would be equally complete if the cereal were taken away. Fortunately, the nutritional breakdown on the side of the box is usually quite complete. Look for high-fiber and low-fat content. With increasing consumer interest in nutrition, such dietary information is widely available.

- Consider making oatmeal for breakfast. Add some cinnamon and raisins and perhaps a little brown sugar and you have a delicious and very filling breakfast that's low in fat. While cooking, you can add flax seeds or bran for added taste and texture.

- Buy boxes of wheat bran and oat bran and add them liberally to other foods. Sprinkle some on your breakfast cereal, or on toast before spreading with peanut butter or jam, and you won't even notice it. Add them to meatloaf or other casseroles, blend them in with the flour when you make muffins or other baked goods, use them to top fruit…. The possibilities are endless.

- Muffins, whether store-bought or made from a standard recipe, can be questionable. Some are low in fat and high in fiber – exactly what you're looking for – while some of the giant ones have over 1,000 calories and are more than 60 percent fat. If it tastes more like a cupcake than anything else, that's what it is. Making your own muffins gives you control over the ingredients and you can seek out low-fat recipes. Many stores are also now offering low-fat muffins – just ask.

- You can't really mix brown and white rice the way you can whole wheat and white flour because they need different cooking times.

If your family really likes white rice, try brown rice with a strongly flavored sauce the first few times. This will help them get used to the new texture and flavor. Of course, you can also cook brown and white rice separately and then mix them together.

- Try other grains that are less commonly used in North American cooking. Barley is great in soups, for example, but can also be used the way we use rice. Bulgur wheat is great in casseroles and as a side dish, or cold in salads. Check out your local health food store or bulk food store for more varieties.

- Pasta now comes in many varieties, not just plain and white. Look for tomato, spinach and whole wheat pastas. All contain more fiber and nutrients than regular spaghetti. Also try couscous, which is a Middle-Eastern version of tiny pasta that cooks quickly and can be served like rice. (Make sure you get the whole wheat version.)

- Most crackers, even the whole grain ones, are pretty high in fat, and they get worse when topped with cream cheese or other spreads. Instead, try plain rice cakes, melba toast or rice crackers. But read the labels carefully – some manufacturers are now producing lower-fat crackers. And watch what you spread on top!

PACKAGED AND CANNED FOODS

This is another area where it's really worth spending a little extra time to read some labels as you shop. Don't be fooled by labels that say "Lite" or "Special diet." Some of these simply mean low in sodium – a good thing, but not something that will help your overweight child. Others may be lower in fat and calories than the regular version, but still not low enough. And plenty of foods are nutritious and low in fat without any special labeling to highlight that fact.

- Some kids love soups; some kids hate them. If your child likes them, encourage him to eat them frequently – research has shown that eating soup can be helpful in weight loss. Of course, you have to pick the right kind of soup – anything with the word "creamy" in the name is probably not appropriate. Minestrone and other vegetable-based soups are a good choice. If you are mixing a canned soup with milk, be sure to use skim milk. If you want it creamier, add a little yogurt. Many companies also offer low-calorie and high-fiber soups, and these can be an excellent choice.

- If you buy TV dinners or other prepared meals, look for the low-fat ones offered by many manufacturers.

- Be careful of rice and pasta that come in packages with powdered sauces (including macaroni and cheese). Most of these are quite high in fat and calories with very little nutritional value. Instead, check out our recipe for homemade macaroni and cheese made with low-fat cheese and skim milk.

- Read the labels on jars of spaghetti sauce and choose low-fat and low-sugar varieties. Or buy plain canned tomatoes and tomato paste and make your own without added fat.

- Salad dressings can be a surprisingly high source of fat and calories. It's self-defeating to serve a low-calorie, high-fiber salad with loads of raw vegetables, only to have it drowned in a high-fat dressing. Fortunately, many brands of salad dressing now come in light and low-fat varieties – make sure you read the labels to be sure they are actually low in fat (remember the 30 percent guideline) and not just lower than a very-high calorie version.

- Canned beans and lentils come in several varieties and are quick and easy to add to many foods without presoaking or other preparation. Stir them into spaghetti sauce or chili, mix them into meatloaf, mash them into a dip – they add protein, lots of fiber and very little fat. Experiment with various types of beans to find some your children like.

FRUITS AND VEGETABLES

This is a great area of the supermarket for going wild. Nutritionists strongly recommend adding more fruits and vegetables to our daily diet. They are excellent sources of fiber and many important nutrients and have minimal amounts of fat. Find out which fruits and vegetables your child likes best and stock up on plenty of them.

- Buy locally grown, seasonal produce whenever possible. It will have the best flavor and will usually be less expensive as well.

- Encourage your child to try new items you discover in your grocery store. Has she ever had persimmon? kiwi? broccoflower? Bring them home and do some experimenting – you may discover a new favorite.

- Try new varieties of foods your child already likes. There are many kinds of apples, oranges, pears, melons, grapes…. Bring home a few of each and compare them. Many of us get in a rut, buying only one type of apple or one type of pear when we could enjoy a much wider variety.

- Go to pick-your-own farms for fruits and vegetables whenever possible. You not only get some very fresh food, you get the exercise of picking what you're going to eat and the pleasure of experiencing a small taste of rural life.

- Some stores offer bags of mixed salad greens already torn in small pieces. If you find yourself too rushed to make salads on many evenings, these can be a real convenience – just add some chopped carrots, green peppers and tomato and you have a great mixed salad.

- The potato is an excellent food with an undeservedly bad reputation. For years, women were told that potatoes (and other starchy foods) were fattening, when in fact it wasn't the potato at all – it was the butter and sour cream used to top it or the oil it was fried in. Potatoes can be quickly baked in a microwave, then cut into small cubes and added to spaghetti sauce; baked and topped with vegetarian chili or salsa and vegetables; boiled and mashed with skim milk and just a tiny bit of butter and prepared in many other nutritious ways. A potato is low in fat, high in fiber (especially the skin) and quite filling – a very good food for someone trying to eat in a more healthy way. A favorite food at Teresa's house is the baked potato sandwich – a hot baked potato is sliced and put between two slices of bread. The bread can be spread with low-fat mayonnaise or the potato topped with skim-milk cheese. Delicious either way.

FROZEN FOODS

The variety of frozen foods available to us today would have been unimaginable even a few decades ago. Freezing has an advantage over canning because no added salt or sugar is needed to make the food palatable, so when fresh fruit and vegetables are not available (or of good quality), frozen ones are often preferable. Many frozen fruits and vegetables taste almost as good as the fresh ones once they've been cooked and prepared.

The manufacturers of frozen foods are also aware of the interest in lower-fat, healthier foods. You can buy low-fat pound cakes, carrot cakes, apple cakes and other desserts in your grocer's freezer; you can also buy entire prepared meals with less than 20 percent fat that heat up in the microwave in minutes.

- Frozen fruit juices can be inexpensive and very good. Be sure you are getting pure juice and not a "juice drink" or "punch" that actually includes as much sugar and artificial flavoring as it does juice.

- Try frozen bread dough for an easy way to have fresh-baked bread with your meals. When bread is hot out of the oven, you can enjoy it without butter (maybe a little jam) and it makes your entire meal seem more special.

BEVERAGES

- Even though soft drinks are low in fat, they have no fiber, are very high in sugar and have little or no nutritional value. It's better to avoid them. Fruit juice spritzers are more expensive but a better choice.

- Don't give your child diet soda, at least not on a regular basis. They simply haven't been on the market long enough for us to know what the long-term effects of aspertame and artificial sweeteners might be.

- Powdered drink mixes are nutritionally equivalent to soda – in other words, they are just sugar and flavored water. It's better to stay away from them.

- Water is the ideal drink. If you are not comfortable with tap water, find a good brand of bottled water and encourage your child to drink lots. One useful rule of thumb: every time he goes to the bathroom, he should have a drink of water. It's also important to drink more water when you are exercising, and your child may notice that she is thirstier as she increases her activity level.

- Fruit juices come in many forms. Always check that the label says pure fruit juice – juice drinks, cocktails, punches and the like all have sweeteners and other ingredients. Try some of the newer blends that mix, say, raspberry and peach juice or cranberry and apple. You can mix fruit juices with plain soda water for a natural fruit "soda" that most children really enjoy.

- Fruit juices can also be frozen in ice cube trays or popsicle makers for frozen treats that replace high-sugar popsicles or high-fat ice cream.

- Try vegetable juices too. While they are not popular with most young children, some like vegetable cocktails, tomato juice or even carrot juice and they're very nutritious.

- Packaged milkshakes are not usually good choices as they tend to be high in fat and sugar. There are, however, some low-fat brands available – read the label to be sure.

More Shopping Tips

- If you have a fruit and vegetable market near your home, try doing at least part of your shopping there. You will find a wider selection of fresh produce, high quality fruits and vegetables and sometimes helpful tips on food preparation.

- Another good place to shop is your local health food store. These stores often have items not available anywhere else, including baked goods, candies and other treats that are low in fat and sugar and contain no artificial ingredients. Yes, prices do tend to be higher, but it's worth making a visit to see what is available and might be useful in your meal planning. Don't assume, however, that everything in the store is low-fat.

- You could also try shopping at a bulk food store for your grains, dried beans and fruits and other ingredients. Buying in bulk means you will usually pay less and these stores often carry unusual grains (quinoa, spelt, etc.) that are hard to find in grocery stores.

- If there are any ethnic stores in your community, they may be worth a visit. Many cultures have based their cuisines on lower-fat and vegetarian foods. Their stores feature foods that may be new to you but will add variety to your meals.

- If you are including meat in your meals, consider buying from a butcher. He or she will help you select lower-fat cuts, trim the fat from chops or steaks and give you suggestions on how to cook the tougher, low-fat meats.

Home Cooking: Cooking Techniques for Low-Fat, Low-Calorie Cooking

Whether you like to cook or cook just because you have to, the techniques you use will have a big influence on the amount of fat and calories in your family's diet.

It is well worth investing in a couple of good, comprehensive cookbooks that will help you learn to cook in new ways and reduce your family's fat intake. If you aren't sure which cookbook will suit your family's food preferences, borrow copies from the library first and try them out. Then buy your own copies of the ones you like best.

GENERAL COOKING TIPS

Use your microwave to reduce the fat in foods. For example, you can brown ground beef in a plastic strainer set over a glass bowl inside the microwave (a pound of meat will take approximately five minutes on high power – be sure to stir it occasionally during the process). The fat will drain through the strainer into the bowl and you will be left with lower-fat meat.

You can also use your microwave to soften onions, green pepper strips, celery slices and other vegetables that are going to be added to a sauce or casserole, rather than having to sauté them in oil or butter. Simply heat them in a bowl for a minute or two.

Avoid frying whenever possible. It always adds extra fat to the foods – sometimes quite a significant amount. Sometimes you can replace frying (of meats, for example) by simply cooking the food in a nonstick frying pan. Or you may be able to brush the food very lightly with oil and bake it in the oven instead.

Follow the USDA Food Guide Pyramid. It recommends five to nine servings of fruits and vegetables daily, and for some of us that's quite a big change. But you will find it very helpful in reducing the fat in your child's diet, because fruits and vegetables are low in fat and high in fiber – exactly what you're looking for.

Getting that many servings each day means that you must be aware of it at every meal. Try to be conscious of ways to add fruits and vegetables to everything you serve:

- Top breakfast cereals and pancakes with fresh or drained, canned fruit.

- Add extra fruit to yogurt.

- Make a "milkshake" for breakfast by mixing skim milk and a banana in the blender (you can add a little orange juice, too, if you like).

- One of Teresa's son's favorite breakfast foods when he was younger was banana mashed together with orange juice and wheat germ.

- Start every meal with a vegetable soup or a salad (it seems more elegant that way, too).

- Grate vegetables into spaghetti sauce, meatloaf, meat pies and casseroles of all types.

- Try cutting the meat in stews in half and doubling the amount of vegetables.

- Top baked potatoes with broccoli or green beans.

- If you've traditionally served one vegetable with your meal at suppertime, try serving two or three.

- Remember that fruits also go well with many entrees.

- Use fruits and vegetables as garnishes and encourage your children to eat them.

- Serve fruit or vegetable juices rather than soft drinks with meals.

- Give fruits and vegetables as snacks throughout the day and before bed.

A friend of Teresa's has a traditional meal that she serves every day during the summer. Because it comes out different every time, we never get bored with it, and yet it's simple enough that it isn't a lot of work.

First, she makes a large salad using whatever greens and raw vegetables she has in the fridge (everyone is invited to help with this). Then she sets out several different breads, buns, pita breads and crackers along with various cheeses, cold meats and spreads. Everyone makes their own sandwiches to go along with the salad. For dessert, she sets out a large bowl of mixed fruit and everyone helps themselves. It's the perfect meal for all those lazy summer days when you don't feel like heating up the kitchen anyway – and, if you are careful about the cheeses and meats you set out for the sandwiches, it's also a low-fat and very nutritious meal.

The moral here is that modifying your diet to help reduce the family's fat intake doesn't have to be a complicated process requiring dozens of cookbooks and new techniques. In fact, the simplest meals are most often the lowest in fat.

School Lunches

For many parents, the school lunch is an incredibly challenging part of the nutritional day.

Mary-Ellen gets up at six-thirty every morning so she can be showered and ready to go when her four children get up for breakfast. While they're eating, she's packing their lunches to take to school: sandwiches, fruit, drinks and a treat. On many mornings she discovers she's forgotten to take a loaf of bread out of the freezer the night before, there is no transportable fruit in the house (her kids say the bananas turn to mush after being bounced around on the way to school) and there's nothing to drink. Sometimes she ends up stopping at a 7-Eleven on the way to school to pick up a ready-made sandwich (cost: $3) and a treat of some kind. She remembers her own school days in England when the school provided a hot, ready-made lunch for every child and wishes they'd do the same thing now.

It seems unlikely that school lunches will be introduced in the near future, so Mary-Ellen's probably going to have to continue struggling with the problem. And it can be especially challenging to pack school lunches for your overweight child – lunches that will fill him up without fattening him up.

Let's look at each aspect of the typical home-packed school lunch.

The Sandwich

- Use whole grain bread. If your child isn't crazy about it, try one slice of whole-grain bread and one slice of white bread, and when he gets used to that, go for all whole grain. Try rye bread, pumpernickel bread, oatmeal bread, bran bread and other varieties, as well as plain whole wheat.

- Try pita bread, buns and other variations on the plain old sandwich. Make triple-decker or pinwheel sandwiches on the days when you have a little extra time.

- Plan low-fat fillings. That means forgetting about most processed meats, nut butters and regular cheeses, as they are all high in fat. Try instead low-fat cheese (made from skim milk), our low-fat yogurt cheese (see recipes) and lower-fat meats such as sliced chicken or turkey breast. There are also some bean-based spreads that can replace peanut butter if your child likes them. (A small amount of peanut butter is not a big problem if it's your child's favorite.)

- Leave off the mayonnaise, butter or margarine. They really add a surprising amount of fat and calories to the sandwich. Many sandwiches are just as good without the high-fat spread. Try mustard, corn relish, ketchup or other flavorings to season the sandwich filling. You can also buy low-fat mayo for those times when you really need some, or mix mayo half-and-half with skim-milk yogurt.

- Sneak in as many vegetables and fruits as you can. Some ideas that have worked with our kids include:

  - Add grated carrots, grated or thinly sliced apple, or sliced banana to peanut butter.

  - Mix orange juice, chopped raisins and grated carrots with low-fat cream cheese or yogurt cheese (it tastes much better than it sounds).

  - Add chopped peaches to low-fat cream cheese or yogurt cheese.

  - Add lettuce leaves to practically everything and put them on both sides of the filling (you can send them in a separate container if kids complain that they get mushy).

  - Add green pepper rings or sliced tomatoes to cheese or meat fillings.

  - Make tuna, salmon or chicken salad with a small amount of mayo/yogurt and mix in chunks of celery, green and red pepper, onion, apple and carrots.

  - Use potato salad (again, made with a mayo/yogurt dressing) with vegetables added as a sandwich filling.

  - Try all-fruit spreads, such as apple butter, peach jam or others prepared with minimal extra sweetening, either alone or with another filling (apple butter, for example, is great with sliced chicken or turkey).

- You can also sometimes replace the bread with a fruit or vegetable:

  - Slice an apple in half, cut out the core, spread with peanut butter, almond butter or low-fat cream cheese and stick the halves back together again.

  - Fill lettuce or cabbage leaves with tuna salad or a similar filling and roll them up. Fasten with a toothpick and wrap snugly before packing.

  – Take two stalks of celery, fill with peanut butter or a low-fat cheese spread, top with raisins and press together before wrapping carefully. Teresa calls this "Ants on a Log" and her kids love it.

THE THERMOS

• A thermos can be a pain (kids are always losing them, leaving them at school or forgetting to give them to you to be rinsed out), but if you are willing to make the effort they can be a big help in planning a filling lunch.

• Use it to send broth-based soups (vegetable, minestrone and lentil are good examples), chili, pasta and sauce and other low-fat, hot dishes.

• It's also good for drinks: low-fat hot chocolate in winter (made with cocoa, sugar and skim milk – easy and delicious), fruit juices or fruit slushies (fruit juice mixed with shaved or crushed ice) in warmer weather.

• Use it to keep a fruit salad or mayo-based salad (like coleslaw) cold and crisp.

OTHER ADDITIONS

• Always include fruits and/or vegetables.

• Raw vegetables are often popular, especially if you can include a small container of low-fat salad dressing or seasoned yogurt to use as a dip. Carrot and celery sticks are traditional and they do travel well, but consider raw mushrooms, cauliflower and broccoli florets, strips of green and red peppers, zucchini strips, chunks of cabbage and any other vegetable your child enjoys.

- Use small plastic containers to send along mixed salads – and don't forget the fork! Send any dressing separately (it will make the salad terribly soggy otherwise) and pack tomatoes separately, too.

- Buy individual servings of canned fruit packed in water or juice. These are expensive but very convenient if your children like them.

- Use those small plastic containers to send along cut-up fruits you prepare yourself such as watermelon or cantaloupe.

- Pack whole fruits carefully. We've never had any luck with bananas or pears – they bruise too easily – but apples, grapes and oranges generally survive the trip.

- Dried fruits (anything from raisins to dried apricots and apple slices) also make good, filling lunch-box additions that are easy to pack.

- Think of carbohydrates if your child complains his lunch isn't filling enough or if she arrives home absolutely starving at four o'clock. Add a container of air-popped popcorn, some pretzels or a low-fat bran muffin, for example.

- Individual containers of yogurt are popular treats and can be a good choice if you choose skim milk yogurt with a minimal amount of sweetening.

- Granola bars sound good and healthy but most are high in fat – the soft and chewy ones usually have more fat than the hard and crunchy varieties. The ones that are dipped in chocolate are basically candy bars. Read the labels before buying!

- Fruit leathers are popular with children, and these are low in fat although many are sweetened with extra sugar. (If your children really like these, it isn't difficult to make your own.)

LUNCHTIME TREATS

What do you do about the question of treats in your child's lunch? You might have eliminated desserts after dinner at home, but can you expect your child to do without when every other child in the classroom is munching on chocolate bars, fudge brownies and bags of potato chips?

Kathy was very concerned about her daughter Karina's weight, so she packed lunches very carefully. Karina got a sandwich with a low-fat filling, a container of salad and a thermos of juice. Kathy thought everything was fine until she volunteered to help out at the school by supervising the lunch hour.

She noticed that most of the other children had chocolate bars, cookies, potato chips or other treats in their lunches, and at first she felt quite smug that Karina's lunch was so healthy and nutritious. Then she discovered that Karina was trading her sandwiches, and even her allowance, for the treats in her classmates' lunches.

"I felt terrible," says Kathy. "I had no idea lunches were so difficult for her."

"I eat my lunch, but I'm still hungry," Karina explained. "And I see all the other kids eating cupcakes and chocolate bars and cookies and I really want some. I'm sorry."

Kathy decided she had to modify her approach. Most of the items she packed would still be low in fat and calories, but each day she would include a treat so Karina wouldn't feel hungry or left out. Kathy set aside some time each Sunday to prepare nutritious treats (see, for example, the chocolate cake in our recipe section). She also visited the health food store in her town and found some low-fat bars and cookies that she could add to Karina's lunch.

"I know she probably trades them for a bag of potato chips sometimes," Kathy says. "But she's concerned about her weight and nutrition, too, so I know she eats her own lunch most of the time. I realized I was going overboard by trying to restrict her so much."

Remember that school lunches are social occasions as well as meals. The child who already feels different because he or she is overweight may want very much to be part of the group by having lunches just like everyone else.

After-School Snacks

Another challenging time for the overweight child is during the hour or so after school ends until dinner is ready. Many children come home absolutely ravenous – it's been a long time since lunch.

Teresa was born in England, and her British parents carried on some of their traditions even after the family moved to Canada. One that Teresa really appreciated was the serving of afternoon tea each day at around four or four-thirty – just the time the kids arrived home from school. Tea, for her family, meant a light meal that was different every day. Sometimes it was grilled cheese sandwiches and soup, sometimes it was a meat pie, sometimes a fruit pie served with custard. This light supper was followed by a bedtime snack at the end of the day. (Her father ate a heavier supper on his own when he came home from work.)

This pattern of eating is actually more helpful to an overweight child than the traditional one. What typically happens is that the child comes home from school hungry, snacks on whatever is convenient (potato chips, leftover birthday cake, cinnamon toast) and then an hour or so later is called for supper. The usual evening meal is quite heavy, but even though the child isn't all that hungry any more, he or she usually eats what is served. This is followed by dessert and possibly another snack before bed – and, not surprisingly, continuing weight gain.

If you can arrange to serve a nutritious and filling after-school snack, followed by a light supper, your overweight child will definitely benefit.

Parents who are at home full time can usually make this change fairly easily, but the parent who is at work when the child arrives home, or who has to arrange for a babysitter during this time, may find it more difficult.

Some possibilities:

- If your child is going to a neighbor's house or an after-school day-care arrangement, pack an extra snack in his school backpack to be eaten when he arrives. This could be a package of dry cereal (let the sitter add milk), a fruit salad, a muffin, and so on.

- If your child is at home alone (or with siblings) for some time before you finish work, make plans the night before to leave a prepared snack. Veggies and dip are always popular, and can be cut up and arranged on a tray, then covered with plastic wrap and refrigerated before you go to bed. They'll still be okay the next day.

- Leftovers from supper the day before can be reheated quickly in the microwave for an easy after-school snack.

- Fill buns with a suitable spread (tuna salad made with low-fat mayo, for example), wrap and place in the fridge.

- Whenever you make or buy muffins, add one or two to a bag that you keep in the freezer. Soon you'll have quite a variety. Then your child can choose one and thaw it out in the microwave when he's hungry.

- Make up a large bowl of fruit salad and keep it in the fridge. (Be sure to add a little lemon juice to the liquid to keep apples, pears and bananas from turning brown.) It will keep well for several days and your child can simply serve himself.

- Another good "keeper" is tabouli, a grain-based salad that can be made from a packaged mix or from our recipe.

- If you are cooking while the kids want to snack, set out the vegetable that you plan to serve for supper and let the kids "sneak" them. Our kids even like eating frozen peas and corn (and they don't eat them cooked).

When you do get home and start supper, you can plan for it to be a bit lighter because you know that your child has already had a head start on the meal.

Meatless Meals

Meats are one of the major sources of fat in our diet, so reducing the amount of meat we eat is an important step in healthier eating. We have already suggested serving smaller portions, but having at least one or two meatless meals each week can also be beneficial.

Miriam's family is vegetarian, and Teresa has several vegetarians in her family who eat no meat at all, as well as one aunt whose family eats no meat or dairy products. We have both tried to develop a repertoire of meatless dishes that everyone in our families will eat (not always easy) and to look for ways of adapting our most popular dishes.

If you simply replace meat with cheese, you probably won't reduce the fat in your diet unless you use low-fat cheese. You need to look for other alternatives. Here are some ideas for making popular dishes into vegetarian variations:

- Many kids are quite happy to eat spaghetti sauce (or any tomato-based pasta sauce) without any meat in it. If it doesn't seem substantial enough that way, try adding TVP (textured vegetable protein, available at many bulk food or health food stores), which has the texture of ground beef. We have also added chopped cooked potato, chickpeas or lentils to the basic sauce for added fiber and protein, and they've all gone over well.

- A vegetarian lasagna is delicious, but most are too heavy on the cheese to be low in fat. Try making it with extra layers of lasagna noodles, using low-fat ricotta or low-fat cottage cheese with chopped spinach mixed in instead of ricotta, topping it with low-fat mozzarella, and adding plenty of grated vegetables to the tomato sauce.

- Pizza can be good with minimal cheese. Use a low-fat tomato sauce for the base, top with sliced tomatoes, onions, green peppers, mushrooms, thinly sliced broccoli florets and sprinkle with a little strongly flavored cheese. After it's baked, use a clean paper towel to soak up as much of the excess oil as possible.

- One of Teresa's vegetarian daughter's favorites is the veggie melt sandwich. This is an open-faced sandwich, best on thickly sliced bread. Toast the bread lightly (in the oven or toaster oven), then top with a selection of cooked and thoroughly drained vegetables (zucchini, broccoli, cauliflower, green peppers, green beans plus raw tomatoes, thinly sliced cucumber, mushrooms). Grate low-fat cheese on top and heat under the broiler or in the toaster oven until the cheese melts.

- Meatless chili is always a hit. You can use TVP to give a meaty texture, or just mix several varieties of beans (Miriam usually uses a can of navy beans, one of kidney beans and one of lentils) with tomato sauce or canned tomatoes, diced green and red peppers, chopped onions and frozen corn. Add enough chili powder and other seasonings to get the flavor you like and cook for 30 minutes if you used sauce or an hour if you used canned tomatoes and their juice.

- Try making a stew without the meat – just lots of vegetables. Your family might not even notice what's missing.

- If you're in a hurry for a quick meal and have decided to mix up a commercial package of macaroni and cheese or other pasta and sauce mix, try cutting the butter called for in the instructions quite drastically. Miriam has made macaroni and cheese with just a tablespoon of butter instead of the quarter-cup listed on the package, and it tasted fine.

- Investigate recipes from other cultures. Most countries have at least some innovative vegetarian meals; some, such as India, have a wide selection of meatless recipes. New flavors and spices make mealtimes fun and your family will be less aware of the lower-fat content.

- Check our recipe section for more easy meatless recipes.

Eating Out with Friends and Relatives

Every adult who has ever been on a diet will recognize this dilemma. You've been careful about what you've eaten all week long, even though it hasn't been easy. Then Saturday comes and you're invited (along with the rest of your family) to your parents' home for dinner. Mom's made all your favorites, including that cheese, beef and heavy-cream casserole that you love, and there's chocolate mousse pie with whipped cream – real whipped cream – for dessert.

What do you do? You know how hurt Mom will be if you don't eat these wonderful things she's prepared, and if you insist on sticking to your diet you know there will be a barrage of questions. How can you handle this?

Your overweight child won't be on a diet, of course, but meals at friends' and relatives' homes may cause problems for him. You don't want him to be rude, but you also want him to continue the new pattern of healthy eating that you are trying to establish.

First of all, let your child know that an occasional high-fat meal isn't a serious problem. If he just wants to eat what everyone else is eating, that's okay. He can get right back into his healthier eating again as soon as he's home, and sometimes fitting in with friends or relatives is more important than minimizing fat and calories.

When you know that the meal is likely to be quite rich and heavy, you could serve a salad or raw vegetables or fruit before you go. This will help fill everyone up and make the higher-fat offerings less tempting.

If the meal is served family-style, with dishes passed around and each person taking as much or as little as desired, or as a buffet, encourage your child to take generous helpings of the lower-fat foods (such as vegetables, potatoes, rice or pasta) and small portions of the higher-fat meats or cheese dishes. He can skip the gravy or other rich sauces, or give himself just a taste.

If the food has been served in pre-assigned portions, your child could just eat small amounts of the higher-fat foods. Don't pressure him to do this, though, because it can be very difficult to resist foods that you really like when they're right there on your plate. If he's urged to eat more by the host or hostess, a comment like "Oh, he had quite a big lunch so he's not too hungry right now" may help.

Imaginary allergies can be useful, too – nobody is insulted by an allergy. Naturally, you don't want your child to actually lie, so she could say, "My mother thinks I might be allergic to dairy products" to avoid being urged to eat ice cream or cheese casserole. It's not exactly a lie – after all, he might be allergic to almost anything at some point in his life. And it may help him out of an awkward situation.

Resist the urge to chastise the relatives about the less-than-healthy meals they're serving, or to proudly announce your family's changed eating styles. It only puts people's backs up and can embarrass your overweight child by drawing unnecessary attention to him.

When you invite people over for meals, offer a variety of nourishing and tasty low-fat foods, and encourage everyone to take as much as desired, without urging them to take more than they feel like.

These occasions are another opportunity for your child to learn skills that will be important to him throughout his life. He'll always be going out for meals and he'll always have to choose the right foods for himself without insulting anyone. With your support and guidance, he can learn to handle these situations in a polite way.

Television

Morning. Aaron wakes up, goes to the bathroom, snuggles back under the blankets and turns on the TV. With any luck, he can get in 15 minutes or more of his favorite show before his dad starts yelling at him to get up. He gets dressed slowly, with his eyes glued to the screen. In the kitchen, he prepares a bowl of cereal then carries it into the family room to watch the rest of his show.

After school, he'll grab a quick snack – a bag of chips or a peanut butter sandwich – and then get comfortable in front of the set again. Like many families, Aaron's eats supper while watching TV as well. Afterward, he does his homework in his room with the set still on for company.

When Aaron's friends come over, they often watch TV together. Sometimes his parents rent movies for the family, or just for Aaron on evenings when they're busy. While they may seem to watch a lot of TV, they really aren't much higher than the North American average of 28 hours per week. As Aaron points out, all the other kids in his class watch a lot of TV, too. Their conversations in the schoolyard focus on TV characters; many of their games are based on acting out ideas they've gleaned from TV plots. If Aaron didn't watch so much TV, he'd be unusual.

The Link between Television and Weight Gain

So if watching TV is so normal, how can it be a problem?

TV isn't a significant problem for some children, although researchers have expressed concerns about its effects on how children learn, respond to violence and behave. In this book, however, we are considering only the relationship between watching TV and body size. Those children who are naturally thin continue to be that way even if they do love TV. But for a child with a tendency to put on weight, TV can be a real hazard, for three important reasons.

One is that research has shown that television-watching significantly lowers the viewer's metabolism. A child reading a book or drawing a picture is burning calories at a higher rate than a child watching TV, even though the reader seems to be just sitting there and as inactive as the TV watcher. In fact, mental activity – such as that required to read a book, or even to sit and think – requires fuel, so calories are consumed. Television, however, seems to involve very little activity on the part of the person watching – it's as though the child's brain is switched off and the information is simply being passively absorbed.

Researchers are concerned that a child who watches many hours of TV may experience an overall lowering of the metabolic rate that will persist even when he or she is not watching TV. (This is similar – but of course in the opposite direction – to the effects of aerobic exercise, which raises the person's metabolism for hours after he or she has stopped exercising.)

A second problem is that the child who is watching TV is not getting the physical exercise that we know is important in maintaining fitness. If you're reading a book and a friend invites you out to play, it's easy to slip in a bookmark and come back to your story at another time. If you're watching TV, on the other hand, the temptation to stay and see the end of the program is almost impossible to overcome. How often have you called your child to come and do something, only to hear the response, "As soon as my show is over"? And TV often becomes addictive, perhaps because it does provide such passive entertainment. Few people will read even the most gripping novel for as long as four or five hours at a time, yet many will watch TV for that long or longer (and admit afterwards that the shows they saw were terrible!).

Because of this, television can use up many hours of a child's time without anyone noticing – time that could be much better spent in other ways to improve the child's health and fitness. When you consider that children usually sleep more than ten hours at night, and probably spend at least six hours at school, plus time for meals, chores and homework, their time for active play is quite limited. To allow television to cut into those hours can mean that exercise is missed out on altogether.

Finally, television promotes eating patterns that are less than healthy. You won't see many commercials for broccoli, pears or other low-fat and nutritious foods. Instead the ads (and particularly the ads on children's shows) try to encourage people to buy highly processed foods that tend to be high in fat and sugar and low in fiber. These are exactly the foods that should be minimized in the healthy diet.

We know these ads work or companies wouldn't be spending millions of dollars annually to have them broadcast into our homes. And some research suggests that people with the tendency to be overweight are more sensitive to the cues the advertisers give them; the sight of delicious-looking food and the encouraging words of the announcer are likely to make them want something to eat even if they're not really hungry.

One researcher also pointed out that the characters on TV programs tend to snack on high-calorie foods and rarely are shown eating a nutritious meal. Yet they are always (of course) *very* thin – giving a very confusing message to the children watching.

It's clear that television can have a significant role to play in the lives of overweight children. But, as in most North American families, yours may rely on TV as a babysitter, a source of entertainment and relaxation or company when others aren't around. Cutting back on TV viewing may seem impractical or too much of a sacrifice. How can you reduce your dependence on the tube and wean your child away from it without too much pain?

Reducing Your Family's TV Time

PREPARATION

Before you try to make drastic changes in your child's TV-watching habits, do some preparation. Television has been called "the Plug-in Drug" and, as with many drugs, it definitely has addictive properties. You can't reasonably expect your child to give it up cold turkey without a fight. Here are some tips to make the process easier:

- Evaluate your current situation. How many hours does the family currently watch? If you have one or more overweight children, what are their TV-viewing patterns? Spend a few days or a week simply keeping track of who is watching and for how long. This information will give you a starting point for any changes you decide to make.

- Educate the whole family. Check your library for one of the many books on the hazards of TV. Discuss the research we have described above about TV's effect on metabolism and fitness. Let them know that you think this might be a problem and that you're hoping to do something about it.

- Be honest with yourself: many parents realize that they have been using the TV as a babysitter to keep the children content and happy while they prepare supper, have a private conversation or relax after work. Other parents find it a useful way to help children wind down before bedtime or to keep them occupied while parents are out at work or elsewhere. If that's the situation in your family, part of your preparation will be planning other ways to fill in those times.

- Enlist as much family support as you can, and decide how to deal with a non-supportive partner if that is your situation. Frequently one parent is eager to cut down or even eliminate television while the other one either isn't convinced that it's a problem or is too attached to favorite programs to even consider cutting down. If this will be an issue in your household, plan in advance how to tackle it. If your partner can't be convinced, maybe he or she would be willing to watch TV in a separate room (perhaps a bedroom or the den) during the times you've decided to have the family set turned off.

EASING-INTO-IT APPROACHES

Try these ideas for gradually reducing the amount of TV time in your family:

- How many TV sets does your family own? The most recent statistics show that many households now have more than one set per person. When Teresa moved into her new house, she discovered that the previous tenants had cable in every single room – no matter where you went in the house, you could watch TV! In that situation, it's hard not to watch a lot of television, because it's always there, always available. If your family has several TVs, one approach to reducing TV watching may be cutting back on the number of sets in your home. Perhaps the extras could be donated to charity or permanently hooked up to the video game set. It's much better to have a single, family TV that everyone has to share, even though you may have to go through more negotiations to work out the best ways of sharing. Think of this as a way of teaching your children social skills.

- Where do you keep the TV? If at all possible, keep TVs out of your children's bedrooms. Because the children are out of sight there, it's easy for long periods of time to go by before anyone realizes that Johnny's been watching TV for hours. And many children will turn the set on quietly and watch it long after you think they've gone to sleep. Don't put your set in the most comfortable location – your best bet may be an unfinished basement or another room less appealing than the family room or living room. You don't want any of those cozy couches and chairs that make TV viewing even more appealing. You can always move the set upstairs temporarily if your family wants to get together for a movie.

- Can you get a small TV or a black-and-white one? It's hard to resist those big-screen sets that dominate the room, but a little set (especially if it's black and white) is much less appealing and easier to ignore. You'll probably sit down and watch it if the show means a lot to you, but otherwise it isn't worth the effort. (These sets are cheaper, too.)

- Could you do without cable? Yes, it does mean missing all those important sports shows and other stuff you watch faithfully, but not having cable can significantly reduce your children's viewing time. If you only get a couple of channels, the chances of there being something on that they want to watch are much lower than if they have the choice of a dozen or more possibilities. One study of a remote northern community showed that obesity rates remained consistently low for many years. However, once cable TV came into town, most of the residents showed sizable weight gains after just one year. There were no other changes in the community – they were just watching a lot more TV.

- Consider investing in a timer. These gadgets attach to the TV and are preset by the parents to allow only a limited amount of television time. It won't go on until the time you have set and it will go off again when you have decided it should. This can be very useful if your children are at home alone for long periods of time while you are away at work or other activities. Remember, though, that some children will figure out how to break into and change the timer in a surprisingly short period of time. And if you have several sets, you will need one for each set, which can get expensive. Joan says, "I found the timer helpful because it eliminated the arguments. Before, I sometimes found myself in a real battle. I'd turn the set off, Jeff would turn it on, I'd turn it off again and Jeff would turn it on again and soon we'd be screaming at each other. Now he might complain, but when it's off, it's off. The timer does it, not me, so he tolerates it better."

- Ration TV viewing. If you've followed our preparation steps, you already have a good idea of how much TV your family watches. Now make a new goal, and don't make it too drastic. Could you cut the TV time by 20 percent? You can accomplish this in more than one way. You might allow a certain maximum number of hours per day or a maximum number per week – if you watch nothing on one day, you can watch more the next day. The key is to control the amount of TV being watched. The biggest risk with this approach is that the allowed maximum becomes the goal – if Joey's allowed to watch three hours of TV per day, he makes darn sure he watches the full three hours, even if the shows aren't that interesting. Be careful not to make too big a deal of this rationed approach.

- Restrict what can be done in front of the TV. A no-eating-with-the-TV-on rule can be a big help in many ways: it will keep your family room cleaner, improve dinnertime conversations and reduce the total time spent watching TV. This rule covers not just mealtimes but snacks, too. One of the identified problems that links TV and overweight viewers is that many people do eat while they are watching. Because their minds are on the TV program and not on the food or any signals their bodies may be giving them, they often don't notice when they're full or not hungry any more. They just continue eating. Television commercials and programs provide plenty of encouragement to eat more, as well. It's also useful in many cases to insist that homework not be done in front of the TV. Your child will concentrate better if he does homework at the kitchen table or at a desk in his room without a TV screen in sight. (Music is a different matter – some research has found that students work better with background music, so let him take a radio with him instead.)

- Let the number of hours the child has exercised equal the number of hours he's allowed to watch TV. This is a different approach to TV rationing, but it has worked quite well in some families. "Max and Seth walk about 40 minutes to school and 40 minutes back, so we count that as exercise," explains Ruth. "That means they can usually watch about an hour and a half of TV each day. If they want to watch more, they can go across the street and play tennis in the park, or go for a bike ride, or bounce on the trampoline down in the basement. Often, though, they get so involved in the activity – like bike riding – that they don't bother coming back to watch TV." Usually this works best if you are fairly relaxed about the exercise requirements. For example, Max and Seth's walk to and from school isn't really vigorous exercise, but Ruth counts it anyway. The idea is to let the children see the importance of having balance in their lives – just as they need to have a balanced diet, so sedentary activities such as watching TV need to be balanced by exercise and more physical activities.

- If you have a fairly large family (this won't work for an only child), assign a TV day to each child. On that day, the child is allowed to watch TV alone without restrictions (other than perhaps shutting the set off for meals and homework times). He picks the programs himself (according to parental guidelines) and can watch for several hours (you may have to place some restrictions here, too). On the other days of the week, other family members have their own TV days, when they can watch individually. So while your child may watch a considerable amount on his or her special day, the rest of the week is TV-free. This approach can require some negotiation to fit around scheduled lessons and other activities, and to accommodate favorite shows. Using the VCR to tape shows that fall on different days can be very helpful; your child may decide to use up all his TV time watching prerecorded shows. If watching TV has been a family activity for you, this approach may be difficult to use, and some children won't like the solitary aspect of it. Children from large families, though, who have endured many battles over which channel to watch and who sits where to get the best view of the set, often like being able to watch without interruption, at least for one evening.

- Begin with small restrictions. Martha was concerned about the amount of TV her son Jared watched, but she didn't want to face the battles that she knew would erupt if she tried to cut him off completely. So she began with small restrictions and gradually increased them. "First, I said no TV before school in the morning," Martha explains. "That wasn't too hard to enforce, because he had a lot to do anyway – getting dressed, eating breakfast and everything. Then I said no TV during meals. We were all used to eating in front of the set so it took some getting used to. Then I said no TV between getting home from school and dinnertime. That's been hard, too, but now Jared's started going out to play during that time. The gradual approach is working well for us." Start by eliminating TV during the easiest time period – a show that nobody really likes, or something that is just a rerun, or a time that's fairly busy anyway. Then try to cut out another chunk of TV time that won't be missed too much. If there is a favorite time – it might be right after school in one family or last thing at night in another – leave that until last, and you may not need to eliminate it at all.

- Emphasize other activities. If you can keep your child busy and involved in other activities, she won't have much time left for sitting in front of the TV set. This can be a real challenge if you are working and your child is alone for any length of time after school. When you aren't there to initiate activities, often watching TV just seems like the easiest thing to do. But you may be able to find a solution. Are there after-school activities she could join (choir, art club, sports)? If you can afford it, after-school care (usually held in the school gym or a local recreation center) might be beneficial even if your child could care for herself at home. Could she help around the house, with food preparation, yard work, other tasks? Are there younger children or pets who need to be taken for walks? Non-TV activities don't always need to involve exercise. Teresa's family loves to do jigsaw puzzles as a group – they especially enjoy the "mystery" ones where, once they finish the puzzle, they have to look for clues to solve the mystery described in a short booklet that comes with the puzzle. This year her oldest son got a 3D puzzle for Christmas – the family is moving on to even higher challenges! Many hours can go by as they gather around the puzzle table trying to figure out where a particular piece goes. Another family activity that has worked well for Teresa and her children is family reading time. They have set aside an hour each evening for everyone to sit together and read silently (when some of the children were younger, Teresa had to read quietly out loud to them while the older ones read to themselves) from any books or magazines they choose. She also has times when she reads aloud to all the children. By doing one chapter a night they've worked their way through many books – including the Narnia series and most of James Herriot's writings. This can take some planning, but it's a very effective approach. When your children become involved in other things, they don't miss TV much.

COLD-TURKEY APPROACHES

Sometimes the gradual approaches to reducing TV watching seem more like a way of prolonging the agony. Every single time you turn off the TV when the daily ration of two hours is up, you're faced with another round of complaining and arguing. You might decide that the best approach is to simply turn off the set altogether.

David's high school class was focusing on a number of environmental issues and each student was challenged to make a sacrifice – to give up something – that would be helpful to the environment. David's choice: to give up television for a month. When he came home with that suggestion, his enthusiasm soon had the whole family involved.

During the first week, everyone was fairly restless. David thought by Wednesday that he'd made a big mistake. He should have chosen to give up eating meat, like his friend Jameel. On

Thursday, though, things seemed to improve. He and his brothers moved past the stage of being bored and started to discover new activities. They also found the house quite peaceful without the constant electronic sounds of the TV set.

When the four weeks were up, all of them were surprised to discover how productively they had used the extra hours that not watching TV had given them. Doing without TV hadn't been as bad as they'd expected. But now the month was over, most of the family was eager to welcome the set back into their lives.

However, going without TV for a month had shown them what changes they wanted to make. They decided to watch just a few shows each week, the ones they had really missed during that month, and to use the VCR to tape ones they really wanted to see. They also made up their minds not to have the TV on while doing other things (eating, doing homework) or just to keep them company.

Why not suggest something similar to your family? The best time to introduce this may be summer, when most of the shows go into reruns and there are plenty of other activities for distraction. It could also be a good New Year's resolution, especially if the children were given plenty of new toys and books for Christmas to keep them busy. Plan a reward of some kind to celebrate an entire month without TV – maybe an outing to a favorite park or recreation area.

Before you start, make plans. What will you do during the time you normally would have watched TV? Maybe a trip to the library to stock up on books or to the Parks and Recreation office to buy a family swim pass would be a good beginning.

Don't be afraid of boredom, though. When your child wanders around saying, "I'm bored," that may just be the prelude to a new creative activity. Give him some time and a little encouragement (comments like: "What do you feel like doing? I'm sure you'll find something"), but let him create his own entertainment. One of the problems with TV is that children who watch a lot often forget how to think up things to do. This will give them a chance to rediscover old interests and try out new ones.

MOVING AWAY FROM TV

It's vitally important that any changes you make in your family's television habits are not seen as a punishment for the overweight child. It's unfair to say, "You're fat because you watch too much television." That's insulting, and probably not true anyway – as we have discussed in previous chapters, weight is a much more complex problem. While television can be a factor, there are many children of average size who watch many hours of TV and don't gain weight.

Overweight children who have suffered a lot of teasing may be more attached to the TV than most. Sometimes it seems like their only friend, a place they can go to be entertained without the effort it takes to communicate with other people or to create relationships. It will be hard for these children to give up even an hour a day without feeling resentful and unhappy. To them, it's a real loss, and they need to know it isn't a punishment or something that's their fault.

If you find your suggestions or attempts to wean your child away from the TV are met with strong resistance, think about the possibility that TV watching may be meeting some emotional needs. Plan to spend extra time with your child and to increase the activities you do together. Make a list of non-TV things he or she likes to do (there are even books available with activities to replace TV – you could buy one and read it together) and see how many you can fit in.

There are many reasons besides concerns about your children's weight to minimize television-watching. We haven't even discussed the problems of exposure to thousands of acts of violence on TV or other issues of program content. Some research suggests that TV is even affecting the ways our children think – or, more importantly, don't think. After many hours of passively absorbing information, some researchers have suggested, children find they are unable to analyze, evaluate and organize things they learn in other ways. It may be that television is not only affecting our children's bodies but their brains as well.

So when you introduce your family to the idea of reducing TV-watching time, make sure you point out the benefits to the entire family. This is not a penance for your overweight child or a punishment the entire family has to endure because one member is overweight. While giving up or cutting back on TV can be a struggle at first, the rewards will be obvious to everyone within a few weeks. Not only will fitness levels go up, but everyone will have more time to accomplish homework and other assignments, take up new hobbies or activities and socialize. Help your children to focus on the things they are gaining, not on what they are giving up.

8

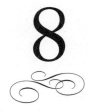

Don't Sweat
the Little Things

Parenting an overweight child can definitely have its frustrating moments.

- Your daughter has been miserable lately because the kids at school have been teasing her about her weight. You sit down for a long talk about the problem and she says she'd really like to change her eating and exercise patterns and lose some weight. You talk to her about food choices and increasing activity, and plan changes for your whole family – starting with walks every Saturday. As you are getting ready for your very first family walk, she says she doesn't want to go – her favorite show is on TV right now.

- You take your son grocery shopping with you and talk about healthy food choices. He helps you pick fruits and other nutritious snacks to load up your cart. But when you arrive home from work the next day, you find him eating a bag of potato chips and a chocolate bar that he bought at the corner store on the way home from school.

- You decide to take your daughter shopping for some new clothes in the hopes that this will boost her self-esteem. But when you get into the store, she wants to buy tight-fitting clothes that only emphasize her chubbiness and refuses to even consider the ones you suggest. You don't want to waste your money buying clothes that you figure she'll wear once, get teased about and never wear again.

- Even though your son hasn't expressed much concern about his size, you really want him to become fitter and healthier. But every meal is turning into a battle, as you try to get him to eat salads and vegetables and he pleads and argues for second helpings of meat and dessert. You suspect he's sneaking food into his room although you haven't caught him yet. Your whole relationship seems to be going downhill.

What can you do when you're faced with these challenges? You want to help your child, but this weight issue seems to be turning into a battle between the two of you.

Remember that your child's self-esteem and your relationship are both far more important than achieving a lower weight. Remember, too, that the only person who can make changes in eating and exercise is your child – you can help, encourage, support, offer suggestions and information, but in the end, it's up to him. Don't let it become your problem, and don't let weight become the reason for conflict between the two of you.

As the title of this chapter says: don't sweat the little things. And compared to the more important issues, being overweight is definitely a little thing.

Expect Change to Happen Slowly

Ask any adult who has tried to lose weight and become fitter: it isn't easy to change established patterns. The changes we have recommended in this book may be small ones for your family or they may be quite drastic; in either case, achieving them may be difficult. It can take a long time to learn to like lower-fat foods and in the process, there may be one step backward for every two steps forward. Finding time to incorporate exercise into your family's schedule can also be challenging, and there may be weeks or even months when you find yourselves returning to more sedentary ways.

But remember that you are not looking at a short-term diet to help your child lose weight (followed by a return to "normal" eating) but at a new – and healthier – way of life. Eating lower-fat foods and exercising every day should be part of everyone's normal routine, and you are trying to help your child onto a road that will lead to a lifetime of fitness. Making the changes slowly helps to make sure they will be permanent. When you think about this longer-term goal, that extra chocolate bar or bag of potato chips doesn't seem like such a big deal.

Making changes slowly is just as important when it comes to exercise. It would be crazy to decide to become fitter and then start out by running a marathon. The intelligent approach is to begin slowly – perhaps by walking for 30 minutes every day – and gradually work up to more challenging exercises – such as running 26 miles, the length of a marathon race. There's a lot of work in between.

In the same way, it's unfair (and even potentially dangerous) to expect a child who has been largely sedentary for years to suddenly become very active. She may need to begin with a daily 15-minute walk or some simple exercises done with a video or to music. Even this gentle beginning might lead to sore muscles the next day and a feeling of discouragement.

The key thing is that some forward steps have been taken.

Don't Let Meals Become a Battleground

This is the same advice that parents of picky eaters are given. For those children, fighting with their parents means they eat less. For overweight children, fighting about food often leads to eating more.

As a parent, your job is to prepare nutritious meals (preferably low in fat) and to serve out the food. That's all. Your job is not to supervise every mouthful your child eats or to be a watchdog counting every calorie.

Your child's job is to decide how much food she needs and what kinds she wants to eat. She will naturally have favorite foods as well as others she doesn't like. You can keep offering the less popular foods and encouraging her to try new things, but don't try to force her. If she's hungry, give her more to eat (more fruit, vegetables, grains, carbohydrates – not an extra pork chop or a bag of potato chips). You won't help her manage her weight or become fitter by making her go hungry – you'll only convince her body to lower its metabolism and increase its signals to get more food.

Don't Make Some Foods "Forbidden"

Remember how tempting the forbidden fruit was in the Garden of Eden? If we make some foods off limits, we make it more likely that our children will crave them, especially if they've already discovered just how delicious ice cream, chocolate and potato chips really are. (We remember one teacher saying jokingly that the surest way to get all children to be readers would be to tell them that reading was absolutely forbidden. He was kidding, but there was definitely an element of truth in his joke!)

Not only does forbidden food seem more enticing, but the temptations children (and adults) face today are much stronger than the few encouraging words spoken by the serpent to Adam and Eve. It's impossible to watch TV, read a magazine or newspaper or listen to the radio without being aware of ads for chocolate bars or the latest snack food. You know that your child will be confronted with these tempting foods every day in the lunch room at school, whenever he visits friends, whenever he steps into a store.

Think how the overweight child feels when she has to watch the other children enjoying foods that she's been told are "bad for her" and "not allowed." If they're so bad for her, why are they constantly advertised – and why do all the other kids seem to be allowed to eat them? Often the overweight child will interpret these restrictions as a punishment unfairly imposed by her parents – and then do whatever she can to get around it.

Diana was an overweight mother whose children were also overweight. Since she was quite young, Diana had been periodically on a diet – first imposed by her mother, and then because she herself wanted to lose weight. She knew that some foods were absolutely forbidden to her and tried hard to keep them out of the house (she made sure her children knew about these restrictions, too), but sometimes she just desperately craved doughnuts and ice cream.

Finally, Diana joined a program for overweight women that emphasized learning to listen to your body's cues. The counselor encouraged her to forget about all the "good" food and "bad" food rules that she'd learned and to simply eat what she wanted.

For Diana, that was quite terrifying at first.

"I knew I'd just go out of control – I'd eat everything. I'd end up weighing 400 pounds."

To her surprise, she didn't. At first she ate lots of doughnuts and chocolate chip cookies, but after a while her body began asking for other foods. Without even thinking about it, she lost some weight and her weight stabilized at this new, smaller size.

"I can't believe how much of my life I wasted obsessing about food," she says now.

She's carried this new approach over to her children as well. When they tell her they're hungry, she asks, "What do you want to eat – what is your body asking for?" and helps them figure out what they need. The children also went through times of eating large amounts of formerly forbidden foods, but now they're much less appealing. A half-full container of ice cream can sit in the freezer for weeks.

This approach can seem frightening to parents. What if your child just keeps on eating large amounts of those fattening foods? You need to recognize that if you forbid certain foods, your child may very well continue eating them, but he will also experience enormous guilt and stress, which is often much more damaging than the physical effects of the foods themselves. While no foods should be forbidden, it's certainly helpful to provide information about nutrition and healthy eating. No foods are truly bad, and you can help your child create a balanced diet that also has room for some purely pleasurable foods.

Preventing Eating Disorders

Anorexia and bulimia were hot topics a few years ago. Every newspaper and magazine ran articles on eating disorders for a while and then the issue faded away from public attention. Many people think that, since the media spotlight has moved elsewhere, the problem of eating disorders has gone away, or at least diminished. They're wrong. They continue to be a major problem with serious consequences for large numbers of teenagers, most of them young women.

What does this have to do with overweight children? Unfortunately, some teenagers who become anorexic were overweight when they were children. They were criticized, strongly encouraged to diet, praised when they lost weight. They believed the myth that "you can't be too rich or too thin." (Anorexia and other eating disorders are complex, and young people become anorexic for complicated reasons. However, this pattern has been singled out by several researchers as one which contributes to the development of this kind of problem.)

One researcher points out that the attitudes overweight children have when they begin to diet – attitudes they are encouraged to develop by those around them – are in fact very similar to the mistaken beliefs of anorexic people: "Fat is disgusting, if I'm fat I'm out of control, I must take control of this problem and lose weight, if I'm thinner I'll be more attractive and more successful." This is often precisely the message that parents and other adults are mistakenly trying to get across to overweight children, but this same message can become extremely dangerous if the child believes it so wholeheartedly that anorexia is the result.

While people often talk about the risks of being overweight, the risks of being underweight are even more serious. Anorexia can be fatal. Even when it isn't, the person may suffer irreversible damage to the liver, heart and reproductive organs that will cause ongoing health problems.

How can you avoid this?

Talk about Getting Fitter, Not Thinner

A thin person may have little muscle tissue, plenty of fat accumulations in the internal organs and little endurance. A very fit person may be quite heavy – we just read a profile of a female aerobic instructor who weighs 182 pounds, yet is very muscular and has tremendous endurance. Increasing fitness should be your goal, not becoming thin.

Don't Equate Attractiveness with Thinness

This definitely goes against the grain in our society, but it's important that children understand that thin people don't have the monopoly on attractiveness or being loved. Take them to the art gallery or borrow an art book from the library and show them the rounded bodies that were considered most desirable only a few generations ago. Point out larger-size people that you see as attractive.

Don't Talk about Your Own Body in a Disparaging Way

You may think that your child doesn't listen to what you say, but that is only when you are telling them what to do. They hear adult conversations even when they look as though they are daydreaming. Many of the five- and six-year-olds who say things like "Oh, I'm so fat" are repeating what their mothers say. We are often shocked by what we hear people say within earshot of their children. If you think you are fat or ugly, keep it to yourself.

Encourage Your Child to Listen
to His or Her Body's Signals

Often people manage to lose weight on low-calorie diets only by forcing themselves to ignore the very clear messages being sent by their bodies. They are hungry but they deliberately don't respond to the signals. This can be a dangerous step along the road to becoming detached from the body's reality. Instead, if your child asks for something to eat or says she's hungry, encourage her to eat. You can help her make nutritious, low-fat choices, but it's important for her to respond to her body's cues.

Avoid Trying to Make Your Child
Lose Weight by Embarrassing Him or Her

Parents sometimes take this approach with the best of intentions. They want their child to find being fat so painful and repulsive that she will do anything to be thin. Despite their good intentions, though, the consequences of being given these messages are very negative. Some children will simply absorb the message that they are disgusting and repulsive and continue to be overweight while hating themselves for it. Others will take the message to heart and become anorexic at great risks to their health. Some may achieve the weight the parents see as desirable, but often at the cost of much of their self-esteem as the child becomes obsessive about maintaining an acceptable weight.

Parenting Goals

Parenting an overweight child is, in many ways, no different than parenting any other child. But you have some extra challenges and your child needs extra support from you.

We encourage all parents to focus on four areas in their relationships with their children; these apply even more to parents of overweight children.

TRUST

One of Teresa's students once wrote a short story based on her most traumatic childhood experience. She'd been called to the principal's office and raked over the coals for some fairly minor offense – an offense she hadn't actually committed. Her teacher had blamed her to keep himself out of trouble. Discovering that teachers lie was bad enough, and she wasn't completely surprised that the principal believed the teacher and not her. What upset her the most was that her parents also believed the teacher's side of the story – they didn't trust her.

Trust is a cornerstone of every relationship, and most particularly the relationship between parents and children. Children must be able to trust their parents to keep their commitments, to love them unconditionally, to care for them. And parents must demonstrate their trust of their children – even while they remember that children will (frequently) make mistakes. Maintaining that relationship is more important than rapid weight loss, even if your child is overweight.

Beth had been working with her daughter Jessica to help her change her eating and exercise patterns. But when she went into Jessica's room to vacuum, she found candy bar wrappers and potato chip bags under the bed. Her first reaction was fury – she wanted to call Jessica in right away for a long lecture. Perhaps it was fortunate that Jess was in school at the time. By evening, Beth had calmed down and thought of some other approaches.

"Jessica," she said, "I was vacuuming in your room today and found some candy bar wrappers. I guess you're finding it hard to change your eating patterns."

Jessica looked embarrassed. "Sometimes I really crave chocolate."

"I know how you feel. Sometimes I crave potato chips. And you know, it's okay to eat chocolate sometimes. I've even got some low-fat chocolate recipes that I could make if you'd like." She hugged Jessica and they went into the kitchen to look for recipes.

If she'd responded to her first feelings of anger, the conversation might have proceeded quite differently:

"Jessica, how dare you sneak chocolate bars into your room. I thought we agreed you'd go on a low-fat diet."

"How dare you snoop through my room!"

"Well, I obviously can't trust you. I'll just have to watch you every minute to make sure you're not eating the wrong things."

But Beth recognized that it isn't possible (other than with an infant) to watch your child every minute to be sure they're eating what you want them to eat. You have no choice but to trust them, so it's important to let them know that you do.

Of course, it's equally important to provide your child with information. Talk to him or her (not in lecture format, but in many short, informal discussions) about what we know about healthy eating, pin up a copy of the USDA Food Guide Pyramid, take your child shopping to discuss the foods you plan to buy but, in the end, trust your child to make the right choices. Sometimes he will make mistakes. It is very hard to change eating habits, especially for a child whose inborn tastes draw him to sweet and fatty foods. Trust your child to do his or her best. Offer her all the help you can give, but let her know she's trusted.

RESPECT

After a quiet half-hour reading through the Parks and Recreation handbook, Alison called Kieran into the room.

"I've decided to enroll you in soccer," she said. "The park where the team practices isn't far away. And you know Noah loved soccer when he was your age."

Kieran stared at the floor. "But Mom…"

"What's wrong?"

"I just don't like soccer."

"Why not? It's great exercise. And we talked about how important it is for you to get more exercise."

"I know, but…"

"And Noah loved it."

Kieran was silent for a minute. "But Mom, Noah's not me. I don't like team sports. I don't like soccer. But I'd like to try gymnastics, if I can."

Alison hadn't meant to be disrespectful toward Kieran, but in her eagerness to find a good recreational activity for him, she'd forgotten to respect his individuality. It's easy for us as parents to believe we always know what's best for our children. Sometimes we do (such as when they want to run across a busy road without looking first) but, especially as they get older, sometimes we don't.

Treating children with respect means first of all respecting their individuality. There is no other child in the world like this one and there never will be. So comparisons are not only unfair, but pointless, and expecting this child to be like another child is just unrealistic.

As much as possible, let your child make the choices that are right for her. If you're looking for a sport or other form of exercise, let the final decisions about what to try be hers. Of course you will be limited by what's available in your community and what you can afford, but respecting her choices will make it much more likely that she sticks with the activity she chooses.

Respecting your child also means a firm commitment to respecting his privacy. Avoid any comments about his weight or changes in eating and exercise in front of friends or even other family members.

Gerald, for example, had invited some friends over after school. Despite the fact that he had discussed eating more nutritious food with his mother just the day before, she came into the kitchen to find him eating cookies by the handful, just like his friends. She was annoyed, but she respected his right to privacy by not saying anything.

Later, when they were alone, she asked him if he would like some help with food next time his friends came over. She offered to prepare some lower-fat snacks that they could share.

Many children who are very self-conscious about their weights don't want even their siblings to know that they are trying to become fitter. They're afraid of being teased and ridiculed, especially if there aren't quick results. You may need to respect their privacy in this area, too, and keep the rest of the family out of things.

AFFECTION

Mario was really struggling with his relationship with his daughter Lily.

"The problem is that she's fat," he said. "There's no getting around it. I don't like fat women. And I don't like to look at Lily the way she is." Lily obviously knew how her father felt. She grew increasingly depressed and unhappy, and her weight continued to rise. Finally both went for counseling.

"When the counselor asked me if I loved Lily, I said 'Of course,'" Mario remembers. "But he pointed out to me that I wasn't showing it to her. She didn't feel loved. And when I really thought about it, I wasn't sure if I did love her. Her appearance really got in the way."

But Mario wanted to love his daughter, even if she didn't meet his ideal of a slender child. He decided to build on that foundation, and rediscovered all the good qualities that Lily had. He also began making a concentrated effort to show his affection for her, because he knew that it is the affection that children receive from their parents and caregivers that lets them know they are lovable, worthwhile people.

There are three important ways of showing affection to our children:

Eye contact. Look your children in the eye. Many studies have shown that people who love each other make frequent eye contact, while those who dislike or distrust each other avoid eye contact. When people look at you directly, you feel noticed and cared for.

This doesn't mean you have to constantly stare into your child's eyes. But it may mean turning off the TV when they come to talk to you so that you can really look at them instead of being distracted by the set. It might mean getting down on your knees so that you can see a small child face-to-face. It might mean eating meals without the TV or a newspaper close by so that you can really look at each other.

One-on-one time. In a large and busy family, it can be a real challenge for parents to spend time with each child individually. But it's also vitally important, even if that one-on-one time is only a few minutes. You might make time alone with a child part of your bedtime routine, or you might plan weekly dates with each child when you go out for a meal together. Sometimes, however, a parent feels less comfortable going out with the overweight child because that parent feels self-conscious about the child's size and worries about what other people might think. You might want to schedule time at home, when you can both just sit and talk.

You may also need to schedule this one-on-one time carefully to make sure each child gets his or her fair share of you. That sounds a bit rigid and unspontaneous, but if you are as busy as most parents are today, it might be necessary. Knowing you have planned a date with her and are committed to keeping it makes your child feel cherished and cared about.

When you do have time with your child, try to keep your attention focused on him. This is not a good time to balance your checkbook or catch up on a little grocery shopping. Let him talk about the things that are important to him. It might be his favorite TV show, a problem he's having at school, his best friend. He might also want to talk about his concerns about his weight. But your role here is to listen, to care, to demonstrate your affection by accepting and taking in his feelings.

Physical affection. It's hard to overemphasize the importance of physical affection in a child's life. Studies have shown that hugging and cuddling is so important to an infant that babies who were raised in institutions and never held or touched often died, even though they were fed, diapered and otherwise looked after. Researchers described the condition of these infants as "wasting away" or "failure to thrive"; although their physical needs were apparently being met, without some affection the babies simply stopped growing and eventually died. Physical affection, it turns out, is also a basic need.

Of course, these babies were in institutions where it was quite easy for staff to carry out scheduled routine care for the children they were assigned without picking them up and cuddling them. This rarely happens in family situations, and even parents who experience difficulty bonding with their children usually provide plenty of touching in their daily interactions with their babies. And if demonstrating your love in this way has not come easily in the past, remember that it's never too late to start.

Your nine-year-old won't die if she doesn't have enough hugs. But she will feel a sense of loss of love that can be very painful.

It can be difficult for some parents, who are strongly influenced by our society's feeling of disgust when it comes to overweight people, to enjoy physical contact with a chubby or obese child. They feel repulsed by fat.

If you feel this way, you may be relieved to discover that giving hugs and cuddles will work despite the way you feel. And you will most likely discover that you can enjoy giving your child physical affection even if she is overweight. You soon become accustomed to a heavier body and learn to feel comfortable with it. This is very important to your child's self-esteem, so it's well worth the effort you may need to make.

What about the child who resists hugs? He needs them, too. He may be reacting to the prejudice he feels because he is overweight and the belief that his body is unattractive and not huggable. Your continued offering of physical affection will demonstrate to him in a powerful way that his body is, in fact, acceptable and lovable.

Does he find hugs embarrassing? Keep them private then, or use pats on the back, an arm draped around his shoulders, a quick squeeze of his hand to demonstrate your affection in a physical way. But don't stop giving them. Even if he seems embarrassed or says, "Oh, Mom, cut it out," he needs those touches. They are as essential as nourishing food and exercise.

CONFIDENCE

Your child needs to know that you have confidence in her, and she needs to develop confidence in herself. It's easy for the overweight child, because of the negative comments she invariably receives from outside sources, to see herself as generally incompetent. After all, if she can't make her weight conform to socially desirable standards, how can she be expected to do anything else well? Many people equate obesity with stupidity and many overweight children have picked up that message.

You can help your child develop confidence in several ways. First, make a point of noting specific accomplishments. Perhaps he did a good job of keeping the baby happy or making her smile while you were busy. Maybe he created a lovely piece of artwork, or helped with a school play, or mastered a math concept that was difficult for him. Make sure he notices these things and don't let him pretend they aren't significant. They are.

Secondly, demonstrate your confidence by giving her responsibility. Perhaps she can prepare supper for the family; if she says, "I don't know how," help her to learn. (There are even cookbooks designed especially for children.) Some parents find it easy to give their children responsibilities; others find it difficult. But when children aren't given these opportunities; they tend to feel incompetent. Yes, they will make some mistakes, but that's part of the learning process. And as they handle situations well, they will develop more self-confidence.

Finally, give your child as many opportunities as possible to try new things. He may be the only child in three generations with musical talent, and if you don't let him try piano lessons, he may never discover it. Learning about new things not only helps children develop learning skills but also helps them feel more competent. Your child's new ability might be as simple as riding a bike or using the family camera to take his own pictures. But learning to master a bike or a camera can be a big step toward developing confidence in his ability to master the next challenge that comes along.

Working on strengthening these areas of your relationship will help not just your child, but you. Parenting an overweight child does have some unique challenges, but it's easier if you can keep the issue of body size in perspective. Working toward fitness goals should not become the only focus of your family's life: there are too many other important aspects of parenting that shouldn't be short-changed.

Appendices

Ten Things
You Should Never Say to an
Overweight Child

1. You'd Be So Attractive if You Just Lost Some Weight

This comment (and many others like it, including "You've got such a pretty face!") is often made with good intentions. The speaker hopes to boost the child's confidence by making a positive comment about his or her appearance, and at the same time give a not-so-subtle encouragement to lose weight.

In fact, though, it is incredibly hurtful. The underlying message is, "but, of course, you're not attractive now." Young children have great difficulty in visualizing future changes and usually find it impossible to act on this statement the way the speaker intends. If the comment has been "You've got such a pretty face," the child always hears the unspoken ending to that sentence: "too bad your body is so ugly."

Overweight children are as beautiful and lovable as any other children. To hurt them with these half-hearted compliments can only damage their self-esteem.

2. If You Weren't So Greedy (or Lazy) You Wouldn't Be So Fat

The research makes it very clear that being overweight is not caused by "personality defects" such as greed or laziness. This comment is simply not true. Any child psychologist will tell you, though, that these kinds of statements tend to become self-fulfilling prophecies. The child who is told often enough that he or she is greedy or lazy often internalizes that comment and begins to believe it – and to behave that way.

What do we mean by "greedy" anyway? Is it a crime to enjoy food, as many children – including, of course, many overweight children – do? Many parents with picky eaters wish their children would have a little more enthusiasm about their mealtimes. And what is "lazy"? Yes, many overweight children would benefit from increasing their physical activity level. So would many thinner children. But most of them aren't lazy – they are simply putting their energy and interest into other areas (perhaps computers, books or television).

Comments like this add layers of hurt. Not only does the child have to deal with the social stigma of being overweight, but now he is accused of greed and laziness as well.

3. No Dessert for You, You've Already Had Enough

This kind of comment is dangerous in several ways. First, it makes the dessert a special, forbidden treat, which naturally becomes more attractive to the child. Anything a child is told he can't have becomes very desirable. He may decide to swipe some later after everyone else has left the kitchen or sneak down in the middle of the night for a treat.

If other people in the family are eating the dessert, the child is placed in a very painful situation. He's being punished for being overweight and being forced to endure watching the others enjoy something he can't have. Can you imagine handing out cigarettes to a group of friends while telling the smoker who is trying to quit that he can't have one? The child's natural reaction tends to be anger and resentment, and often, again, a determination to steal or somehow acquire the food that was forbidden.

Finally, by making the decision that the child has had enough, you are stopping her from listening to her own body. She needs to let her body signal her when it's full and as long as you tell her, "No, you've had enough," she won't be listening to her inner cues. Then how will she know when to stop eating when you're not there? It's better to ask, "Are you still hungry?" and let her respond depending on her body's signals.

If this is an ongoing problem in your family, you may need to change your approach to dessert. Try planning fruit or pudding-based desserts that are low in fat and high in nutrients, so they become a valuable part of the meal. Then everyone can enjoy them without any concerns. If you do choose to serve a rich dessert, it should be offered to everyone, and perhaps the rest of the meal could be kept fairly light (a main-dish salad, for example) to compensate.

4. If You Lost Some Weight the Other Kids Wouldn't Tease You So Much

If that were true, only overweight children would ever be teased. In fact, kids are always finding something to tease other kids about, whether it's wearing glasses, haircuts, clothes, stuttering, doing unusually well or badly in school, and on and on. Yes, overweight children are often teased by other kids, but you need to make it very clear that this is not the overweight child's fault. She does not deserve teasing and humiliation because of her size (which is what the comment above seems to imply). Would you tell a child who wore glasses that if he'd improve his eyesight he wouldn't be teased?

If teasing is a serious problem for your child, this might be a good time to approach a teacher at school about helping children learn better social skills. It is never appropriate to make fun of another person's body, whether it is because they are skinny, disabled in some way, a different race or overweight. Our society's bias against larger-size people is so strong that children are often permitted to say these things in front of teachers and other adults when we would stop them immediately if their comments were racist or directed at disabled people. Overweight children deserve just as much consideration.

5. You Probably Wouldn't Have Hurt Your Leg (Pulled a Muscle, Sprained an Ankle, Twisted a Knee) If You Weren't Overweight

Is this true? Possibly. There is some evidence that overweight children are at slightly more risk of injury during activity, although it may be caused by their inexperience in sports rather than their weight. But it's also true that many thin people are injured during activities from sports to shoveling the driveway after a snowstorm.

Even more important, you need to look at the likely effects of this comment. Your child is probably not going to think, "Yes, Mom's right, I should lose weight somehow so that I'll be less likely to get injured playing sports." Instead, his reaction will more likely be: "Fine, I won't play baseball [or soccer or whatever the activity was at the time he was injured] ever again." Instead of promoting health and fitness, this kind of statement actually encourages him to become less active.

The overweight child who is injured while playing sports or engaged in any other activity needs the same reassurance and support that any other athlete would get. Help her learn the skills she needs to play safely and reduce the risk of injury, but don't link it to her weight.

6. I Don't Think Light Colors Are a Good Choice for You – How about This Nice Dark Brown Dress?

If your child likes the dark brown dress, there's nothing wrong with that choice. But if your child prefers the bright red or the light green, let her express her tastes in her clothing.

Too often overweight children are encouraged to stay in the background of life, and dressing them in dull, dark clothes is one way of trying to make them less noticeable. Some shy children would prefer that anyway, but other children, whether they are larger than average or not, want to be center stage, and dressing brightly can be part of that. Respecting their choices is very important.

These arguments over clothes can often be a reflection of the parent's discomfort with the child's size. You are choosing dark clothes because you want him to seem smaller. But it's much more important that he feels comfortable with his body – and if a bright red sweater makes him feel cheerful and powerful (even though you feel it draws too much attention to his plump figure), then it may be very valuable to his self-esteem for you to let him wear it.

7. Only Thin Kids Can Do Gymnastics (or Ballet). Why Don't You Sign Up for Piano Lessons Instead?

There's nothing wrong with piano lessons. But if your child is interested in gymnastics, dancing, swimming or any other activity that's traditionally associated with thinner people, please don't discourage her.

Too many adults have the idea that only thin and talented people are entitled to dance or play sports. Most children haven't discovered that concept yet, and the longer we can keep them from believing in it, the better.

Sometimes parents say this to protect their child from future hurts. If Charles signs up for ballet, they worry, he'll be teased by the other children and end up feeling worse. Yes, teasing is a concern for overweight children – but he might just as easily be teased by the other kids at his piano lesson. He may, instead, find a new group of friends linked by a common interest in dancing that overrides their differences in body shape and size.

In other cases, the parents are concerned about their own embarrassment. They cringe at the thought of watching chubby Jessica running across the gym floor or swinging from the bar in a tight leotard, or seeing Derek's round tummy over the top of his swimming trunks. Those feelings are the result of the indoctrination we've received about how "disgusting" it is to be heavier than the average, and they can be very destructive for parents with overweight children. Some parents have to work very hard to overcome this feeling and be able to watch their overweight child walk across the beach in a bathing suit and not feel uncomfortable about how he or she looks.

We know how important exercise and activity are in everyone's life and any involvement your child has is a positive thing, even if you think the sport is not entirely suitable. Try instead to respond in a positive way: "I think it's great that you're interested in gymnastics. Let's see if you can try a few classes to see if you like it."

8. After You Lose Weight, We'll Go on a Holiday (or Buy You a New Bike or Any Other Reward)

Setting up weight loss as a goal for a child is a terrible mistake. First of all, children should seek to maintain their weight until they grow into it, rather than actually losing pounds. If the reward is desirable enough, you may find the child embarking on a dangerous low-calorie diet that can damage her health and start her on the road to a lifelong struggle with weight. Even then, she may not be able to achieve the goal you have set for her (read our chapter on the causes of overweight to understand why).

This approach also starts a pattern that can be difficult to break. Far too many overweight adults put their lives on hold "until they lose weight." How many people have you heard say, "When I lose weight, I'll buy some new clothes." "When I lose weight, I'll join that club I've always wanted to be part of." "When I lose weight, I'll take that vacation to Florida." Time goes by, the weight stays the same and the person has missed out on a great many things she really wanted to do.

If you follow the tips in this book and your child becomes fitter and healthier, that will be reward enough. As you are making these changes in your family's lifestyle, encourage your child to do things he likes. He deserves to enjoy life! If he himself suggests, "I'll do that after I lose weight," try to encourage him to do it now.

9. If You Want to Lose Weight, You're Just Going to Have to Stay Hungry Most of the Time

Reread the earlier comments – children should not lose weight but stabilize until they grow into it.

Staying hungry, though, is never a good plan for weight management. When you are hungry, your body responds in several ways. It sends increasingly strong signals to let you know that it needs food (signals that are especially hard for a child to ignore). Even more importantly, it slows down your metabolism to use any food you take in more efficiently. Overweight children generally have fairly slow metabolisms to start with; low-calorie diets simply slow them down even more. While they may, in fact, lose some weight this way, it is quickly regained.

Children who are hungry most of the time tend to become completely focused on food. They think about it all the time, and they are more likely to give up and binge on their favorite treats.

Instead, encourage your child to eat a healthy, low-fat diet with the emphasis on carbohydrates, fruits and vegetables, and to eat enough that he feels comfortably full. Help him to recognize his body's cues that tell him when to stop eating. If he's still hungry, he should eat more – but he should choose his foods from the low-fat items mentioned earlier.

This gradual moving toward healthier eating will help your child find the most appropriate weight for her body and maintain that weight.

10. Your Problem Is That You Just Don't Have Any Willpower

Your overweight child has just as much willpower as anyone else (or just as little as anyone else!). As we have discussed elsewhere in the book, weight is much more complicated than simply a lack of willpower. Again, these comments tend to be self-fulfilling prophecies. The child quickly becomes convinced that he doesn't have any willpower, that he's likely to give in to any temptation (including, perhaps, drugs and alcohol) and since no one offers any suggestions on how to increase willpower, he follows the expected pattern. When high-fat treats are offered, he takes several – what else would you expect from a person with no willpower?

In fact, the heaviest people are likely to be those with the most willpower – the people who have dieted, lost weight, regained it, dieted again, regained the weight, dieted again and so on. Their metabolism is now so slow that they must eat very few calories just to keep from gaining even more. This cycle is very difficult to break out of once it has been established.

What if your family has been working on changing your eating patterns and then you find your child has pigged out on rich chocolate ice cream? Don't condemn him for his lack of willpower. This is a good time to talk about tastes and to discuss how difficult it is to keep to a healthy diet when so many high-fat foods are around. You might try to buy a lower-fat substitute for the food that tempts him the most strongly. Reassure him that occasional binges or overindulgences in treats are not failures or reasons to give up altogether.

Suggesting that a child has no willpower is the result of believing another of the myths about body size: that being overweight is somehow the result of a moral deficiency. It isn't. A person's character and worth as a human being are not related to body size. It is more important for your child to grow into an adult who can recognize his innate worth and value his strengths than for him to grow up as a thin person.

APPENDIX 2

Ten Easy Ways to Reduce Fat

1. Serve smaller portions of meat and choose lower-fat meat products (such as extra-lean ground beef). Trim off any visible fat.

2. Serve fewer eggs. In baking, you can often replace one egg with two egg whites.

3. Try frozen yogurt instead of ice cream, but check the label; names can be deceiving, but the ingredient list is accurate. Better yet, make your own.

4. Spread jam or fruit butter on bread instead of butter or margarine.

5. Top baked potatoes with salsa or low-fat mayonnaise-type dressing instead of sour cream and butter.

6. Use skim milk instead of whole or 2 percent.

7. Serve low-fat and high-fiber muffins instead of cupcakes, danishes or other baked goods.

8. Remove the skin from chicken before serving – that's where most of the fat is. You don't have to remove it before cooking. This just dries out the chicken.

9. Buy tuna packed in water, not oil.

10. Serve low-fat cheeses and low-fat yogurt.

Ten Tips for Eating Out

1. Do It!

Sometimes when you are worried about your child's weight and about eating healthier foods, eating out seems like too much of a challenge. You'd rather just have all your meals at home, where you can control how they are prepared, how large the portions are and what ingredients go into the "secret sauce."

But eating out is important for several reasons. First, it's part of most children's social lives – the other kids are going to McDonald's and Armadillo's and it's hard for the overweight child to feel left out of those activities. He or she (perhaps even more than children of average size) needs to participate in the social events other kids are involved in.

Secondly, even if you decide not to eat in restaurants or fast-food places for several years, at some point your child will need to deal with these situations. It may happen in junior high when he and his friends go out for lunch or when she is taken to a restaurant by a relative, but at some point we all have to learn to make good choices in restaurants and to deal with the array of food that is presented to us. It's much easier if you can teach these skills while your child is still young and you are there to help with the choices.

Finally, eating out adds an element of celebration to mealtimes that is also socially valuable. It can be a pleasant break for the adult who is doing most of the cooking and perhaps an introduction to new foods for the children. So even though there are challenges to eating out with an overweight child, the benefits definitely outweigh the drawbacks.

2. Try Ethnic Restaurants to Get to Know Foods from Different Cultures

While our North American approach to cooking sometimes seems to be based on the "let's fry everything" philosophy of food, many other cuisines are based on lower-fat ingredients. Of course, in many restaurants the original recipes have been modified to suit North American tastes. Look for more authentic Japanese, Spanish, Italian, Vietnamese and other restaurants to get a taste of the real thing.

Will your children eat couscous or curry? They may surprise you – children will often eat things in restaurants (or at other people's homes) that they wouldn't touch if you made it for them yourself.

Tina and her husband can't afford to take their three children to eat out very often. They decided that when they do, they'd like it to be an event. So each month, Tina chooses a different country (one that has a restaurant near their home, if possible, although they have occasionally traveled quite a distance to get to more unusual dining spots) and does some research about the foods normally eaten there. She involves the children in this project, too, and they check books out of the library to learn more about their country-of-the-month: a little geography, history, maybe some art or music. Tina may even try preparing some of the foods at home, if they don't look too difficult, but the highlight is the family's visit to a restaurant to sample authentically cooked foods.

Of course, eating at ethnic restaurants doesn't mean that every item on the menu will be low-fat and high-fiber. You will, as always, have to read over carefully and make appropriate choices. But it may expose your children to some interesting new tastes and ways of preparing food, and demonstrate convincingly that delicious meals don't need to be the traditional meat-and-potatoes combinations many of us are used to.

3. Sit-Down Restaurants May Be More Expensive Than Fast-Food Places, but Their Selection of Healthy Food Is Often Larger

Fast-food chains build their reputations on a simple, basic approach. They serve predictable food quickly – and that means they necessarily have a very limited range. Offering only a few items on the menu allows them to be fast and efficient. Most specialize in burgers; a few feature chicken or fish but these tend to be battered and fried (turning a fairly low-fat food into a rather high-fat meal).

To succeed, they also need to focus on the most popular foods and these are, most often, the higher-fat ones. The current interest in healthier eating has brought salads, lower-fat burgers, low-fat shakes, muffins and a few other changes into the fast-food chains, but many have been phased out again because the average customer still prefers the regular burger with fries and a soft drink.

These realities mean that fast-food eating is a bit more challenging for you than a regular, sit-down restaurant might be. In some places (Taco Bell is one example) there is almost nothing on the menu that would fit into the low-fat guidelines.

To help you in these situations, you might consider buying a copy of a small booklet called *The Low-Fat Fast Food Guide* by Jamie Pope-Cordle and Martin Katahn and published by W.W. Norton & Company. It tells you the fat grams, fat percentages and other nutritional information about the foods served at the country's top fast-food chains.

A sit-down restaurant will usually have a wider selection on its menu, so you can choose items that minimize fat and maximize fiber and carbohydrates.

4. Start with a Salad
– but Be Careful about the Dressing

It can be a very useful policy to always start your meals with a leafy garden salad. Salads offer plenty of fiber and lots of nutritious vegetables that will help fill you up, and they are available almost everywhere – even fast-food places usually offer salads now.

The problem, of course, is that the salad dressing is often very high in fat. One package (a single serving) of McDonald's ranch dressing, for example, contains 20 grams of fat; one package of Arby's ranch dressing has 38.5 grams of fat. Some places offer a low-fat variety – always ask about it. (McDonald's "lite" vinaigrette, for example, has only 2 grams of fat – a very significant difference.) Try your salad without dressing at all (Teresa has learned to prefer it that way) or use some corn relish, low-fat yogurt or salsa as a tasty topping. You can also ask for a lemon or lime wedge to squeeze over the salad. Always ask for the dressing on the side so that you can add as little as you want.

Not all salads are created equal, either. Caesar salad is very high in fat (a shame, because so many kids like it). Potato salads, creamy coleslaw and pasta salads all rely on high-fat mayonnaise-based dressings for flavor, and that same dressing makes them high in fat.

If you are going to begin with a garden salad, have it served first, before the rest of the meal arrives. Otherwise your child may set the salad aside and fill up on the other food, then not have room for salad. It's healthier if she fills up on salad and doesn't have room for the mashed potatoes and gravy later.

If salad isn't your child's favorite, start with a soup – but not a creamy one. Some kids love soups and some kids won't touch them. If your children like them, they can be a good alternative to salads to begin a meal. One researcher found that people who ate soup tended to be fitter and weigh less than people who didn't. The catch is that they must be broth-based soups, not creamy ones. Some good options: minestrone soup with plenty of vegetables, pasta and beans; onion soup (ask for it without the cheese); lentil soup; beef and barley. A hearty soup can, in fact, be a whole meal.

5. Use Salad Bars and Buffets Wisely – To Add a Variety of Low-Fat Vegetables and Starchy Foods Like Potatoes, Rice and Breads to Your Meal

Buffet meals can be your child's downfall if he's determined to try the lasagna, the pork chops, the fried chicken and the sausages. Instead suggest choosing one entree, and filling up the plate with vegetables, potatoes (preferably baked or mashed, not fried), rice, bread and fruit. Handled properly, the buffet can be a good way to get more variety into your meal rather than more fat.

What if your child wants to go up for seconds? You can ask, "Are you still hungry?" and encourage her to listen to her body's signals rather than just having more because it's there. If she is genuinely hungry, allow her to take second helpings (especially if everyone else is), again with an emphasis on vegetables rather than meat and cheese.

6. Try Eating Vegetarian

You might not want to become full-time vegetarians, but skipping the meat when you're eating out is one way of reducing the fat. Instead of basing your meal on meat, you can enjoy a variety of vegetables and carbohydrates that will nourish you and fill you up.

Try one of the many vegetarian restaurants that exist in most large communities. Or visit any restaurant but choose vegetarian foods (remember that if you simply substitute cheese for meat, you probably are not reducing fat).

This approach can be challenging, but many children find it fun to go through the menu and pick out the vegetarian choices.

7. Leave Off the Special Sauces, Cheese, Gravies and Whipped-Cream Toppings

Those sauces and toppings seem so innocuous that it's hard to imagine they actually contain large amounts of fat – as much as 15 or 20 grams per serving – even though only small amounts are used. If your child will eat a hamburger instead of a cheeseburger, for example, he'll cut the amount of fat almost in half – from 19 grams to 10 grams. Or order your french fries plain to dip in ketchup or salsa, rather than drowned in gravy or cheese (one ounce of gravy – a small serving – has 8 grams of fat).

If your child has "bought into" a lower-fat diet, tell him about the fat content of these toppings. Could he enjoy his Big Mac without the special sauce? Is a fruit salad almost as good without whipped cream? Most restaurants are quite prepared to leave off the extras if you ask them.

8. Consider Making a Meal of Appetizers if Main Course Portions Are Too Big

Some of the best meals Teresa's family has enjoyed in restaurants came about when they decided not to follow the usual routine of appetizer, main course, dessert. Instead, they ordered several appetizers – two or three per person, depending on portion sizes – and shared them around a bit. Everyone had more variety in their meal and no one was left feeling stuffed.

Of course, appetizers need to be chosen carefully, with an eye on the low-fat, high-fiber guidelines. But that can often be easier to do from the appetizer menu because there isn't the emphasis on large portions of meat that you'll see in the entree section. Be creative and put together a nutritious but different meal.

9. Aim for Balance

Can you go to a restaurant – fast-food or otherwise – and tell your child, "No french fries, no dessert, no meat"? Perhaps you can, but it wouldn't be very successful. Your child may decide on her own not to order those items, but it needs to be her decision.

Instead, aim for balance in the meal. If your child is longing for french fries from McDonald's, order a small serving but suggest that she balance them with a salad, low-fat muffin, a small burger (rather than a Big Mac) and a low-fat milkshake or fruit juice to go with it.

You may have to think of balance in a larger perspective, as well. Let's say you've been out to a ball game with your child and she asked for a jumbo hot dog and a large order of fries. This is standard baseball-park fare and perhaps, for her, the food is part of the magic of the game. Ball-park vendors don't offer salads and plain baked potatoes, so it's the hot dog or nothing.

What can you do? If you buy her the hot dog and fries, help her to balance it out over the next day or so. It might be good to follow this with a vegetarian day – no meat at all – with an emphasis on fresh fruit and vegetable salads. And next time you go to the ball game, bring some low-fat snacks to enjoy. But you might have to buy a hot dog anyway.

10. Share a Special Dessert with the Whole Family

There are low-fat desserts that can be eaten without worrying about having too much fat in your daily diet. But sometimes what everyone wants is that gooey, chocolatey, rich and very high-fat dessert that this restaurant is famous for.

One solution? Order the dessert with enough spoons and dishes for everyone to share. That way you'll all get a taste but nobody has too much.

Another approach? Have a salad without dressing, then skip the entree and just enjoy the dessert. This wouldn't do for everyday eating – you'll miss too many important nutrients – but if your child is just dying for that special dessert, make that the meal instead of trying to find room for it after a big dinner.

Above all, enjoy your meals out and let your child enjoy them as well. Even in fast-food places, it's possible to make good choices that will meet your child's nutritional needs and keep his overall fat intake within reason.

APPENDIX 4

Holidays and Special Occasions

There are only a few holidays that aren't in some way associated with high-fat, sugar-loaded food – Yom Kippur and Ramadan come to mind. Generally, the year is packed with the other kind:

Birthdays (celebrated with cake, ice cream and bags full of goodies).

Valentine's Day (chocolate; heart-shaped cookies).

Easter (more chocolate; a big ham dinner; Easter breads and hot-cross buns).

Passover (cakes made with ground nuts and millions of eggs; kugel).

Summer picnics (featuring potato salad, fried chicken, hot dogs and the like).

Rosh Hashanah (taiglach, honey cake).

Hallowe'en (bagfuls of candy).

Thanksgiving (another feast of turkey, stuffing, pumpkin pie).

Chanukah (latkes with sour cream; doughnuts; caponata; other fried foods).

Christmas (the biggest feast of all – cookies; chocolate; turkey with all the trimmings).

Those are just the standard holidays celebrated by Christians and Jews, but the holidays of most other religious groups also include special foods and feasting. Sure, Christmas only comes once a year, but with all the other celebrations (not to mention birthday parties) holidays can easily become obstacles along the road to healthier eating. How can you make these special occasions less hazardous to your family's nutritional goals?

BIRTHDAYS

- Try a breakfast birthday party instead of one featuring lunch or dinner. (This will also save you from listening to your child ask at least one million times, "How long until the party starts?") You can serve low-fat pancakes with a variety of fruit toppings, plus fruit juice, yogurt and perhaps a selection of dry cereals and muffins as well.

- For a later-in-the-day party, put out plates of cut-up raw veggies and dip or cut-up fruit and dip instead of bowls of potato chips when the guests first arrive.

- Serve Face Sandwiches and Goofy Salads (see our recipe section) – two easy and nutritious low-fat meals that kids think are fun to eat.

- Try a make-your-own pizza meal. Buy small round pizza crusts (or use English muffins or pita bread cut open), top with a thin layer of tomato sauce and then let the kids put on their own toppings from the selection you have laid out. Forget the bacon, sausage and pepperoni; offer them chopped green peppers, chopped onions, thinly sliced tomatoes, sliced mushrooms, blanched, drained and sliced broccoli and cauliflower, sliced zucchini and any other toppings you can dream up. (Teresa personally hates pineapple on pizza, but if your kids like it, go ahead.) Then sprinkle with a layer of low-fat shredded cheese and pop into the hot oven. Baking time will depend on the type of crust you are using. The pizza crusts will take about 10 minutes; toppings on a pita bread may be ready in just 2 or 3 minutes.

- Serve either cake or ice cream, but not both. Or you can buy an ice cream cake from many ice cream stores, which gives you something to stick the candles in. If you decide to serve cake, consider carrot cake, apple cake or banana cake – or the chocolate cake in our recipe section. And try ice milk or frozen yogurt instead of a richer ice cream.

- Be creative with your goodie bags. One treat (such as a candy bar) is nice, but there are plenty of other little gifts that could be included: sugar-free gum, pencils and pens, pencil sharpeners, stickers, collectible cards, and so on.

- When your child is invited to a birthday party, don't make a big fuss about what she's going to be eating. Let her enjoy herself without worrying that one meal will make her fatter. It won't. You can serve a low-fat breakfast and lunch, and give her a nutritious snack just before she goes, but let her relax and have fun with her friends.

VALENTINE'S DAY

- It's the heart shape that's the key here, so think about other things that could be cut with your heart-shaped cookie cutter. What about using white and whole wheat bread and filling hearts cut out of one piece into the middle of the other? Makes a unique and intriguing sandwich.

- If your child receives a box of chocolates, encourage sharing with others. Remind everyone in the family that Valentine's Day is supposed to be about expressing love, and help them find other ways of showing people that they care.

EASTER

Has hunting for chocolate eggs – followed by eating as many as possible – been an Easter tradition at your house? You might want to consider some changes:

- Hide small gifts instead of chocolate. These can be anything from toys, craft items and jewelry to socks, underwear and new clothes. Have each child search in a different room so they find the things that belong to them.

- Try an outdoor scavenger hunt (in your backyard or a nearby park) and have the items found turned in to you for prizes (and minimize the chocolate). This is more exercise as well as fun.

- Try a follow-the-clues hunt. Each child is given a different clue to solve at the beginning. This clue leads him or her to the next clue, which leads to the next clue and so on until the prize (perhaps one chocolate egg and some new clothes) is discovered. You can make the hunts easier for younger children and as tough as you like for the older ones. Teresa's kids love this – the prize at the end isn't nearly as important as the search.

- If your family traditionally celebrates Easter with a big meal, see our Christmas section for some tips on making it healthier.

PASSOVER

- Fried matzoh can be made in a pan sprayed with a low-fat spray (instead of butter or oil). Use two egg whites and one whole egg for every two servings (instead of all whole eggs).

- Matzoh is the perfect vehicle for butter, but don't slather it on. Put a thin layer on half a matzoh and put the other half on top.

Summer Picnics

Most of us look forward to eating outdoors whenever possible once summer arrives. Unfortunately, many of our favorite summer meals tend to be very high in fat. Here are some ways to make them healthier:

- Many families' favorite things to barbecue – hamburgers and hot dogs – are high in fat. You can improve them by making the burgers out of extra-lean ground beef and making small patties and by looking for low-fat hot dogs in the grocery store. Offer generous toppings of tomato slices, onion and green pepper rings, lettuce, salsa, etc. Buy whole wheat buns to put everything on.

- Better meats for barbecuing include chicken, shrimp, scallops and fish steaks.

- Remember that lots of vegetables are great barbecued. Often a barbecued meal ends up focusing entirely on the meat; be sure yours is better balanced than that.

- Potato salad can be just as tasty but a lot lower in fat if you use low-fat mayonnaise or yogurt instead of regular mayonnaise. Add chopped celery, onions, green peppers and serve with lettuce; leave out the hardboiled eggs.

- Bring fresh fruit for dessert and skip the pies and cakes, or make our low-fat chocolate cake.

Rosh Hashanah

- Focus on the importance of family customs and observances, rather than on food.

- The apples dipped in honey at the beginning of the meal might tame everyone's appetite a bit.

HALLOWE'EN

- Would your children skip going out altogether if you hosted a Hallowe'en party for them and their friends? Perhaps this could be organized by a church group or school. Keep the focus on the fun of dressing up and serve nutritious foods related to the season or the party theme: pumpkin muffins, apples carved as jack-o'-lanterns, and so on.

- Spend time carving a pumpkin, bobbing for apples, decorating your front porch, even if you don't have a party. Move the focus away from the food.

- When your children do go out, send them door-to-door with the smallest container possible; when it's full, they have to come home.

- If they *do* go door-to-door and come home with loads of treats, plan how they're going to be eaten. One parent tells her children they can eat as much as they like that night and then she throws everything else away. They tend to feel pretty sick that evening, but then it's over. Another parent stashes away all the candy and puts one treat in each child's lunch until it all runs out. (It usually lasts until Christmas.) Others ration out a few candies each day to be eaten as dessert after supper.

- Tell your child he must brush his teeth every time he eats a candy or chocolate. This will help to cut down on all-day-long snacking.

- Ask your child to pick out her favorite treats and get rid of the rest (you can always put them in the freezer and give them out yourself next Hallowe'en). Otherwise many children will eat all the candy, even if it's things they don't particularly like, just because it's there.

- Make sure the things you give out at Hallowe'en are nutritious and low in fat. Consider stickers, pencils, small packages of crayons, gum, toothbrushes (one dentist on our street always gives toothbrushes), sunflower seeds, raisins, popcorn. Then if you have some left over, you won't mind your children getting into them!

THANKSGIVING

Traditionally, this is an occasion for eating until your stomach hurts. But it doesn't have to be that way.

- Plan an after-dinner walk. That will encourage people not to eat so much that they can't move.

- Consider having a Pioneer Thanksgiving Dinner, cooking things the way the pioneers might have. That means no fancy sauces and plenty of hearty vegetables and whole grain breads. Serve it by candlelight and talk about the lives of the early settlers.

- Or try a vegetarian Thanksgiving with stuffing but no turkey. It's still delicious. Many vegetarian cookbooks have menus for festive meals.

- Make Thanksgiving an opportunity for sharing. Serve a plain meal of beans and rice, then take the money you might have used for a more elaborate feast and donate it to the food bank.

CHANUKAH

Greasy foods are the mainstay of Chanukah and they can be difficult to avoid. Here are some tips that may help you cut down on fat without feeling deprived.

- Bake your latkes rather than frying them. Put a small amount of oil into a large glass pan and put in the oven for 10 minutes while your oven is warming to 375 degrees. Then spoon your latkes in individually, turning them when they are crisp on the bottom.

- Use either low-fat yogurt or a mixture of sour cream and low-fat yogurt instead of plain sour cream on the latkes.

- Use a sugar cookie recipe that is low in fat and cut out menorah and dreidl shapes.

CHRISTMAS

For those who celebrate it, this is probably the most challenging holiday of all. Besides the big family feast on Christmas Day, children are faced with visits to relatives (with food always being offered), parties at school and with friends, chocolates in their stockings, and on and on. Teresa's children once went through three Christmas dinners: one with her on Christmas Day, one with their father and his family on the following day, and a third when relatives arrived from out of town on December 27. And of course, Christmas dinners are traditionally high in fat and sugar. No wonder most adults end up making New Year's resolutions to lose weight.

How to resolve it?

- Think activity when you're giving your child Christmas gifts. If she's shown any interest in a sport or other form of exercise, look for a gift that will make it easier for her to participate.

- When you're the hostess, serve low-fat snacks and treats. Fresh fruit, attractively arranged with a tasty dip, can be set out on a tray instead of chocolates and cookies.

- Try serving various breads (including rye, oatmeal, whole wheat, carrot, banana, applesauce, lemon) with jams or fruit spreads instead of cookies or crackers and cheeses.

- At Christmas dinner, emphasize vegetables rather than high-fat foods. Serve small portions of meat and higher-fat items such as stuffing, but offer several vegetables.

- Be careful of drinks as well. Eggnog and milkshakes are usually quite high in fat. Try cranberry juice mixed with ginger ale or other fruit juices. Make hot chocolate from skim milk.

- If you're serving turkey, remember that you don't have to roast and serve an entire turkey. Look for leaner cuts, such as the skinless turkey breast roll available in many stores.

- Christmas can be a time for sharing, too. If your family has been given boxes of cookies, chocolates and candies that you really don't need, pass them on to a women's shelter or another group that might find them a real treat.

KWANZA

Some of the Christmas tips are helpful for this African-American cultural festival, celebrated from December 26 to January 1. Try emphasizing substantial salads over fried dishes. Have a look at the black-eyed pea salad and the low-fat yam pie featured in Appendix 5.

OTHER CELEBRATIONS

What do we do when we want to celebrate an anniversary or an achievement? Often we go out for dinner or buy a favorite food. That may be the pattern in your family. But it's important for your overweight child to learn other ways of being rewarded or of celebrating.

Josie remembers: "I don't think my parents did it deliberately, but every time we did something well, we got food. If I got a good report card, we went out to dinner. If I was well behaved in the store, I got a chocolate bar in the car on the way home. When my brother's team won a game, we all had ice cream afterward."

But as Josie grew older she realized that this pattern had become a problem for her. When she was feeling down or discouraged and wanted to give herself a boost, food always seemed to be the answer. And carrot sticks just didn't do it. Instead, she usually went for the chocolate or ice cream treats that had been part of her childhood rewards.

What are some alternative ways of rewarding children?

- A card, a banner across the living room (MIKE HIT A HOME RUN), a note on the fridge (don't put it in a lunchbag – other kids will read it and may make fun of your child). Something in writing is often a good acknowledgment of an achievement.

- Hugs and kisses are always good.

- Plan an outing for the whole family – to celebrate the last day of school, for example, or the end of summer. Maybe you could hike through a local conservation area, go swimming at the nearest pool, go window-shopping at a mall in another city, tour the museum.

- Don't forget books and magazines as rewards – they last longer than food, too.

- Help each child keep his own "I want" list – and when he's accomplished something you want to reward, pick an item off the list.

Think about helping your child find pleasures every day that don't involve food. There can be pleasure in exercise, in spending time with friends, in reading a new poem, in listening to music. Sometimes children in a hurried society, relying on TV for entertainment, are unaware of those pleasures. Help them to discover them.

It isn't reasonable or realistic to expect your child to avoid all chocolate bars or cheesecakes. Instead, by emphasizing low-fat, high-fiber foods, you make it possible for him to eat in a healthy way while still enjoying his treats in moderation. It's a way of eating that can – and should – continue for the rest of his life.

Some Recipes to Get You Started

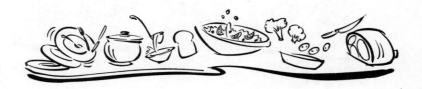

Breakfast

TERESA'S FAVORITE FRUIT SALAD

This recipe is very flexible and you can add any other fruits that you enjoy. Frozen blueberries are good but will turn the apples and bananas blue. Try canned pears or canned pineapple instead of peaches, or other kinds of melon instead of cantaloupe.

If you would like a topping, plain yogurt is delicious. Or try it with vanilla or butterscotch ice milk as a dessert.

1 10-oz. can sliced peaches in juice (or 2 fresh peaches)

1 banana, sliced

1 can mandarin orange slices (or 3 mandarin or clementine oranges)

2 apples, not peeled, diced

1/2 cantaloupe, diced

1 small bunch of seedless green grapes

Pour both canned fruits – with the liquid – into a large bowl. Add other fruits and mix. Let stand for at least one hour or overnight.

Makes 4 servings.

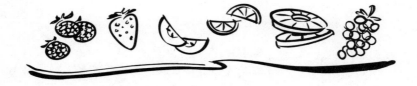

BAKED BANANAS

This is delicious but very easy. It's best made in a toaster oven because heating up the large oven seems wasteful.

◆

1 banana

1 tbsp. lemon juice

1 tsp. brown sugar

Peel the banana, cut in half and slice lengthwise (you will have 4 pieces). Sprinkle with lemon juice, then with brown sugar. Bake in toaster oven at 400 degrees for 4 or 5 minutes until edges brown slightly. If you do this in the microwave instead, it may be somewhat wetter.

Makes 2 servings.

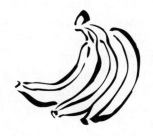

LOW-FAT PANCAKES

1 cup whole wheat flour

1/4 cup all-purpose flour

1/4 cup oatmeal

2 tsp. baking soda

1 tbsp. brown sugar

3 egg whites

1-1/2 cups sour milk or buttermilk (or 1 cup skim milk mixed
with 1/2 cup yogurt)

1 tbsp. plus 1 tsp. vegetable oil

1 tsp. vanilla extract

In a large bowl, mix together the flours, oatmeal, baking soda and sugar. In another bowl, combine the remaining ingredients and mix thoroughly. Add to dry ingredients and mix just until all are moistened. It will still be a bit lumpy. (You can make this the night before and keep in the refrigerator until breakfast time.) To cook, heat a nonstick frying pan over medium heat and spray lightly with a nonstick cooking spray. Pour about 1/4 cup of batter into pan for each pancake. Cook until small bubbles appear on the surface, then turn over. Remove when no more steam appears.

You can add fruit to the batter (blueberries, bananas, raspberries and chopped apples are all delicious) or use fruit as a topping. Or use orange juice instead of the sour milk and add a little orange peel.

Makes 12 pancakes (4 servings).

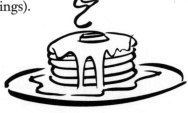

SMOOTHIES

1 cup skim milk

1/2 cup skim milk or low-fat yogurt

1/2 cup or more frozen fruit (strawberries are the best)

1 banana (can use fresh or frozen)

1 tbsp. honey

1 tbsp. bran (if you think of it the night before, let it soak in the fridge with the milk)

Blend everything except the frozen fruit in the blender, then add the fruit one by one while machine is running. You can also add 2 ice cubes if it isn't cold enough.

Makes 2 servings.

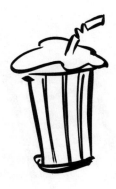

BREAKFAST OR LUNCH SPREAD
(CREAM CHEESE SUBSTITUTE)

1 tub of skim or low-fat yogurt
(a brand that has no added gelatin or thickeners)

Put a coffee filter into a strainer or line the strainer with a few lay-ers of cheesecloth. Place strainer into a bowl that is big enough so strainer won't touch liquid. Put yogurt in filter and place the whole thing in the refrigerator overnight. In the morning you will have a thick spread for sandwiches remaining in the strainer.

Seasonings can be added to the yogurt before the process (oregano and basil, cinnamon and ginger, cumin and turmeric) but you may want to try a small batch just in case the kids hate the sea-sonings. You can also use this in cooking to replace sour cream.

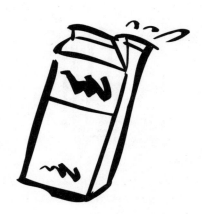

Main Dishes

Two Basic Low-Fat Spaghetti Sauces

1. A LIGHT-TASTING SAUCE

A favorite in Miriam's household

1 28-oz. can tomatoes
1 small onion, chopped
1 bay leaf
1 tsp. dried basil
a few shakes of pepper

Microwave onion for 45 seconds on high and put in a pot. Add tomatoes and their juice and mash them. Add other ingredients and simmer for 30 minutes.

Makes 4 servings.

2. THE TRADITIONAL SAUCE

1 28-oz. can of plum tomatoes, chopped (keep the liquid)
1 6-oz. can tomato paste
1/2 cup water
2 tsp. oregano
1 tsp. sugar
1 tsp. garlic powder

Mix all ingredients together and simmer over low heat for 20 to 30 minutes. Serve over cooked spaghetti or other pasta.

Makes 6 servings.

These are both very plain sauces but many kids prefer them that way. You can add any vegetables you like without affecting the fat content. Or try any of the following low-fat variations:

SPAGHETTI SAUCE WITH POTATO AND SPINACH

To either basic sauce add 1 onion, chopped and cooked for 45 seconds in the microwave, and 1 grated carrot. Then bake a potato in the microwave for 4 minutes, dice into small cubes and add to the sauce. Add 1/2 of a small package of frozen chopped spinach and heat for about 30 minutes. The potato makes the meal seem much heartier.

SPAGHETTI SAUCE WITH BEANS

Take ingredients for either sauce and place in blender container. Add 1 small can of kidney beans and blend until smooth. Add 1/2 can cooked lentils and heat over medium heat for 20 minutes.

SPAGHETTI SAUCE WITH VEGGIES

To either basic sauce add 2 small grated zucchini, 2 grated carrots, thinly sliced celery, 1/2 chopped green pepper, 1/2 chopped onion and 1/2 cup thinly sliced mushrooms. Simmer for 20 minutes.

SPAGHETTI SAUCE WITH TUNA

To the veggie sauce add 1 can of tuna packed in water, drained thoroughly. Simmer for 20 minutes.

SPAGHETTI SAUCE WITH MEATBALLS

If your child really craves some meat with his spaghetti, try making meatballs instead. Because the meat is more noticeable, you can serve a bit less. Use any of the sauces above and make meatballs from 1 pound of extra-lean ground beef mixed with 1/4 cup skim milk, 1/4 cup rolled oats, 2 slices of whole wheat bread torn into small cubes and 1 tbsp. steak sauce. Mix thoroughly and shape into meatballs. Cook on rack in microwave for 10 minutes, rotating rack after 5 minutes. Serve with sauce and pasta.

PIZZA

You can vary this recipe as you like, adding mushrooms, pineapple or other ingredients. Stay away from pepperoni, bacon, sausage and other high-fat ingredients, and be cautious with the cheese.

◆

1 pizza crust

1/2 cup low-fat traditional spaghetti sauce

1/2 green pepper, chopped

1/2 onion, chopped

1 cup broccoli florets

2 tomatoes, thinly sliced

1/2 tsp. oregano

1/2 tsp. garlic powder

1/2 cup to 1 cup shredded low-fat cheese

Spread sauce on pizza crust. Place pepper, onion and broccoli in a small bowl, cover with plastic wrap and heat in microwave for about 45 seconds on high power or until vegetables are soft. Spread on pizza. Top with sliced tomatoes. Sprinkle with oregano and garlic, then with shredded cheese.

Bake at 425 degrees for 8 to 10 minutes or until cheese is bubbling.

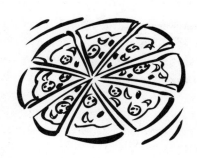

POTATO SUBS

For each sub:

    1 submarine roll, split lengthwise

    green pepper rings

    chopped onion

    one potato, baked and hot

    1 slice low-fat processed cheese

    low-fat mayonnaise or dressing

Spread the sub with mayonnaise and top with cheese. Slice the potato (don't peel it) and arrange on top of cheese. Top with green pepper and onion. Eat while the potato is still warm.

    You can add lettuce and tomato if your children like them. This is delicious, low-fat and very filling.

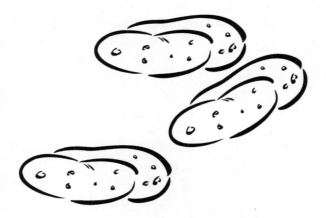

FRENCH FRIES

4 large potatoes, not peeled, sliced like french fries

2 tbsp. olive oil

2-1/2 tbsp. water

Preheat oven to 375 degrees. Mix oil and water in a bowl. Add potatoes and toss until well covered. Arrange on a baking sheet so they don't touch. Bake for 20 minutes, turn them over and bake for another 20 minutes. Sprinkle with salt and serve immediately.

Makes 4 servings.

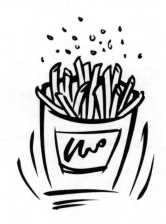

BLACK-EYED PEA SALAD

3 15-oz. cans black-eyed peas

2 cups cubed cooked chicken or turkey

1 cup chopped celery

1 large green pepper, seeded and chopped

1 medium onion, chopped

1 tsp. yellow mustard

1/2 cup low-fat mayonnaise

1/2 cup fat-free yogurt

salt and pepper to taste

Drain the canned peas and put them in a large bowl. Add the other ingredients and mix well. Chill thoroughly before serving.

Makes 4 servings.

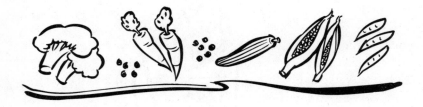

Desserts

CHOCOLATE CAKE

1-1/2 cups flour

1 cup white sugar

1/3 cup cocoa

1 tsp. baking powder

1 tsp. baking soda

1/2 tsp. salt

1 tsp. vanilla

1 tsp. vinegar

1 tbsp. melted butter or margarine

1/2 cup applesauce (homemade or bought)

1/2 cup lukewarm low-fat yogurt mixed with 3/4 cup lukewarm milk

Preheat oven to 350 degrees. Cut out a piece of waxed paper the same size as the bottom of a 9" x 9" pan. Place it in the pan and lightly grease the sides of the pan. Sift the dry ingredients together. Beat in the liquid ingredients (by hand or with an electric mixer). Pour into pan and bake for 30 to 35 minutes, until toothpick tester comes out clean. Cool in pan for 5 minutes and then turn onto a cooling rack. Sprinkle with powdered sugar before serving.

CHOCOLATE PUDDING

This makes a creamy and delicious pudding that can easily be changed. Add almond extract instead of vanilla, for example, or some peppermint extract for chocolate mint flavor.

Or leave out the cocoa and have a plain vanilla pudding that is great over fresh fruit (for example, bananas, raspberries or peaches).

Or, again with the cocoa left out, substitute lemon juice for the vanilla and add a little grated lemon rind – a lemony pudding that is also very good with fruit.

◆

2 cups skim milk

1/4 cup brown sugar

3 tbsp. cornstarch

2 tbsp. cocoa

1 tsp. vanilla extract

In a saucepan, heat 1-1/2 cups of milk and the brown sugar to simmering point over low heat. In a cup or small bowl, mix together the remaining 1/2 cup milk, the cornstarch and the cocoa until thoroughly blended. Add to hot milk, stirring constantly until thickened and starting to boil (2 or 3 minutes). Remove from heat and add the vanilla. Spoon into serving bowls and chill.

Makes 4 servings.

BREAD PUDDING

This is good hot or cold and can be topped with maple syrup or more fruit.

◆

4 egg whites

2 cups skim milk

1/3 cup brown sugar

1/2 tsp. vanilla

4 or 5 slices of bread, cubed

1/3 cup raisins

1/4 tsp. cinnamon

1/4 tsp. nutmeg

Mix together egg whites, milk, sugar and vanilla. Mix in bread cubes, raisins and spices. You can add additional fruit if you like at this point (try 1 apple, grated, or 1 cup of diced peaches). Pour into an 8" x 8" inch baking pan that has been sprayed with cooking spray. Set this in a larger pan that is filled with water to a depth of one inch. Bake 40 to 50 minutes at 350 degrees or until pudding is set.

FROZEN FRUIT DESSERT

Peel and cut up one banana or other soft fruit (peach, mango, a handful of strawberries, etc.) per person. Freeze fruit on a cookie sheet for about an hour (longer is fine). Put fruit in food processor and process until smooth. (There is a point at which it seems this won't work, but it will. Don't be discouraged.) Serve immediately, plain or with hot fudge sauce (see recipe).

HOT FUDGE SAUCE

2 tbsp. cocoa powder

2 tbsp. brown sugar

1 tbsp. confectioner's sugar

1 tsp. corn syrup

1/4 tsp. vanilla extract

1/2 tsp. butter

1 tsp. milk

Mix all ingredients in a 1 cup measuring cup. (The butter doesn't have to mix in completely.) Microwave for 15 seconds, then stir. Microwave for another 15 seconds, watching closely. Remove cup from microwave as soon as ingredients come to a boil. (You may need a few more seconds, depending on your microwave.) Spoon over homemade frozen yogurt or frozen fruit dessert.

Makes 4 servings.

FRUIT WITH DIP

Dip:

> 1 cup low-fat yogurt
>
> 1 tbsp. brown sugar

Sounds simple and it is. Just mix together – it's surprisingly good. For another variation, add 1/4 tsp. powdered ginger.

Serve with assorted fruits:

> sliced apples (dipped in lemon juice)
>
> sliced peaches
>
> sliced bananas (also dipped in lemon juice)
>
> sliced kiwi
>
> diced melon
>
> strawberries
>
> grapes

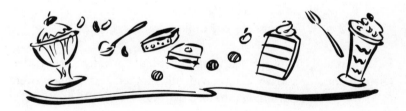

YAM (SWEET POTATO) PIE

Piecrust:

> 1 cup Grape Nuts cereal
>
> 1/4 cup apple juice concentrate (thawed but not diluted)

Mix together cereal and concentrate, and pat into a thin layer on bottom and sides of a 9" pie pan. Preheat oven to 350 degrees. Bake for 8 minutes. Let cool.

Filling:

> 2 medium yams
>
> 1/3 cup sugar
>
> 3 tbsp. cornstarch
>
> 1/2 tsp. cinnamon
>
> 1/2 tsp. ginger
>
> 1/4 tsp. cloves
>
> 1/8 tsp. salt
>
> 1-1/2 cups skim milk or soy milk

Peel yams and cut into cubes. Steam over boiling water until tender (30 to 40 minutes). Mash and mix with other ingredients. Preheat oven to 350 degrees. Pour filling into piecrust, and bake for 35 minutes.

Makes 6 servings.

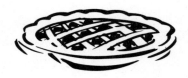

Further Reading

Berg, Francie M. *Afraid to Eat: Children and Teens in Weight Crisis.* Hettinger, ND: *Healthy Weight Journal*, 1997.

Ikeda, Joanne P., and Naworski, Priscilla. *Am I Fat? Helping Young Children Accept Differences in Body Size.* Santa Cruz, CA: ETR Associates, 1993.

Kleinman, Dr. Ronald E., Jellinek, Dr. Michael S., and Houston, Julie. *Let Them Eat Cake! The Case against Overcontrolling What Children Eat.* New York: Villard Books, 1994.

Shaw, Judith B., and Kwiterovich, Peter. *Raising Low-Fat Kids in a High-Fat World.* San Francisco: Chronicle Books, 1997.

Index